Interviewing and Patient Care

Interviewing and Patient Care

ALLEN J. ENELOW, M.D.
Professor and Chairman Department of Psychiatry
Pacific Medical Center University of the Pacific

SCOTT N. SWISHER, M.D.
Professor and Chairman Department of Medicine
Michigan State University College of Human Medicine

New York OXFORD UNIVERSITY PRESS
London Toronto 1972

Sixth printing, 1978

Library of Congress Catalogue Card Number: 72-87036
Printed in the United States of America

FOREWORD

The broadening of the definition of health from absence of disease to the condition of optimal well-being has come at a time when there is a growing national consensus that access to those services helping people to achieve health is a right which belongs to all citizens. It also comes at a time when we have begun to realize that achieving and maintaining health are functions of the entire range of genetic, biological, social, and environmental factors which impinge upon living people. The tasks confronting the health professions have consequently proliferated.

Various professional and sub-professional categories, each concerned with more or less specific segments of patients' lives, bodies, physiological functions, or disabilities, make up what is customarily called the health care team, although the organization of this conglomerate group into something functioning as a team has rarely occurred. In any case, one by-product of these developments has been confusion as to the role of the physician in this emerging system. Is the concept of the physician as society has known him any longer viable? Is his role becoming fragmented into several specific technical functions? If the physician in the future is to have a group of health professionals in his office including nurses, laboratory technicians, social workers, and physician's assistants, what aspect of his traditional role does he delegate, and what does he retain as his own special skill?

Doctors Enelow and Swisher indicate their position on this issue clearly; namely, that the central role of the physician, regardless of specialty or personal interest, lies in his capacity to deal directly with his patients in productive, therapeutic relationships. To form such relationships the physician must be able to communicate effectively. This communication is a continuing two-way affair, in which the physician accumulates information and at the same time generates confidence and understanding. The result of this interaction should be a relationship of mutual trust and confidence, which should in turn lead to intelligent cooperation from the patient in the interest of his own health. Though this fundamental task is shared with other health professionals, it must not be surrendered if medicine wishes to play a leadership role in the increasingly complex health team.

In traditional medical education, the learning of interviewing skills by medical students has all too often been left to chance, with the hope that somehow students would learn them within segments of the curriculum devoted to history taking, physical diagnosis, or clinical specialties. That real success in this aspect of medical education has not been universal seems evident from the proliferation of malpractice suits and the crescendo of public dissatisfaction with the impersonal nature of much medical care received, however well satisfied people may be with its technical quality.

In the College of Human Medicine at Michigan State University a primary curricular precept was established from the beginning: that professionalization of the student in developing effective relationships with patients is at the core of all clinical learning experience from the first term of the first year through final specialty clerkships in the last year. Beginning with simulated patients, aided by closed circuit television and instant replay arrangements, and progressing to real patients with health problems of increasing complexity, students find that interviewing technique is emphasized throughout their undergraduate medical education.

While much of this kind of learning of professional behavior is currently accomplished through personal involvement, there are principles of proven validity capable of being learned and described, and it is this material which is presented in this book. Much of it is in use in conjunction with the physician-patient relationship sequences at Michigan State University.

The authorship of this book is worthy of note, comprising as it does a psychiatrist, and an immunologically oriented internist-hematologist, with major contributions by a sociologist. This effort, then, represents a fusion of behavioral, biological, and clinical science which neatly characterizes the composite role of the physician.

Andrew D. Hunt, M.D.
Dean, College of Human Medicine
Michigan State University

PREFACE

This is not a book on history taking, even though the authors believe that a primary goal of the interview is to gather data. But the traditional emphasis in medical education has been on *what* data to get, and not on *how* to get it. We are interested in what data to get, how to get it and how to synthesize these data into an understanding of the patient's total situation. Interviewing is the principal tool used by the health professional to accomplish this, and is, therefore, a skill which the effective health professional must master. This book is designed to present the principles that will help the learner to acquire or improve that skill. While some of the chapters will be most useful to the medical student, most of the chapters, we believe, will be useful to students of all the health professions.

The roots of this book go back to research on interviewing in continuing education programs for physicians and to the teaching of interviewing to practicing physicians, residents and medical students at the University of Southern California. The collaborators in those undertakings were an internist, Douglas L. Forde, M.D.; a sociologist, Leta McKinney Adler, Ph.D.; a psychologist, Murray Wexler, Ph.D.; and a psychiatrist (Enelow). The first output of this team was a series of programed instructional films on interviewing, developed by Enelow, Adler and Wexler under a contract with the Bureau of Health Manpower, Division of Physician Manpower (contract number PH108-66-202).

In 1967, the collaboration between the authors of this book began at Michigan State University. Working with medical students and planning the new medical school with an emphasis on early introduction to patients and to interviewing led us to the decision to write this book. The planning meeting, in November, 1968, included Murray Wexler, Leta Adler and the authors. The writing began about a year later and has taken more than two years.

Many people have contributed to this final product. Of these, special mention should be made of Leta McKinney Adler, who reviewed most of the chapters and made many helpful contributions to both style and content, in addition to being author of one chapter and co-author of another. The contributions of Drs. Ray E. Helfer, William B. Weil and Mary Ryan on interviewing children; and that of Cyril M. Worby, M.D. on interviewing families, are gratefully acknowledged. A number of members of the Departments of Medicine, Psychiatry, and Human Development at Michigan State University have read selected chapters of this book and have offered many useful suggestions which have been incorporated. Many medical students at Michigan State have read chapters three, four, five and six and have responded to questionnaires about them that were most helpful.

Throughout this project we have had the support of Andrew D. Hunt, Jr., M.D., Dean of the College of Human Medicine, who is responsible for having established an atmosphere in the medical school that made it the appropriate germinal center for a book like this one.

There cannot be a book like this without many hours of hard work in typing, re-typing, collating the manuscript and shepherding it through review by many colleagues. Since a number of chapters went through as many as eight drafts, this task was not inconsiderable. Our special gratitude goes to Mrs. Shirley Hurni who supervised it and Mrs. Debbie Coats who did much of the typing. Doris Saenz, medical illustrator, MSU Medical Media Center, contributed to the design of the cover. Indexing was made possible by the careful help of Lisa Kearns, Patience Enelow, and Abigail Enelow.

In many ways this was a collaborative project of faculty and students of Michigan State University with the authors. The student was the audience for whom it was written, and it is the Michigan State University medical student to whom it is dedicated.

East Lansing, Michigan A. J. E.
June 1, 1972 S. N. S.

CONTENTS

Interviewing and Patient Care

1

THE INTERVIEW IN CLINICAL MEDICINE

1 INTRODUCTION

Diagnosis and treatment in medicine begin with the interview. Gathering information, evaluating it, discussing the findings with patients, planning, and monitoring treatment all depend on interviewing. The greater the skill of the interviewer, the more complete and reliable will be the information on which he bases his diagnosis. A skilled interviewer will succeed in transmitting findings to the patient so that they are clearly understood, are not unduly frightening, and inspire trust and confidence in the physician. Skilled interviewing affords the possibility of involving the patient in the planning of his treatment, making it much more likely that he will carry out the doctor's recommendations. A good doctor-patient relationship requires effective interviewing and increases the likelihood that the physician will be able to monitor progress in treatment as well as to get early information about developing complications. Finally, good interviewing is the basis of the positive side of health care that is so often sought in vain by patients: that the physician not limit his help to the removal of discomfort but that he seek to produce a state of comfort and a feeling of well-being. Clinicians are likely to consider the term "medical interview" as synonymous with what is called history-taking. The medical interview is much broader than that.

Failure to follow good interviewing principles will often result in an inaccurate diagnosis or a significant gap in the information needed for planning treatment.

A fifty-three-year-old widow with a long history of anxiety, many somatic complaints without discernable physical basis, and frequent visits to her physician consulted him because of chest pain of several days' duration. As usual, she was quite worried about her new symptom. The physician interviewed her briefly, asking a few highly specific questions. After a somewhat hurried physical examination he noted a slight reduction in blood pressure and assured her. "You're just fine, Mrs. D. We've talked about your worries and fears before. That's all it is." That night she was taken to the hospital by ambulance. She had a myocardial infarction, which was now manifested by severe, crushing chest pain, and a marked drop in blood pressure. Because the range of information elicited during the interview that afternoon was limited the physician was unable to arrive at an accurate diagnosis.

A thirty-three-year-old divorced secretary with known hypertension was interviewed at a psychosomatic case conference. The Senior Resident in medicine brought her to the conference as a complicated management problem because her blood pressure could not be kept under control with any of the usual anti-hypertensive medications. He had an excellent and detailed account of all of her physical difficulties and the complications of her hypertension. He described her as a cooperative patient and had found nothing of psychological significance. The interviewer began with an open-ended query: "What kind of troubles are you having?" With great heat the patient replied, "Men!" She went on in a torrent of emotion, sometimes angry, sometimes weeping, to describe difficulties with her employer, her ex-husband, her father, and now with male friends and lovers. She talked about her use of alcohol in large amounts to control her alternating anger and depression. All of this was new information to the resident, who had interviewed her in a highly structured, directive-interrogative manner.

When a patient consults a physician he expects of that physician that he find the sources or causes of discomfort and that measures be taken to remedy the disorder. To accomplish these things, the physician's first task is to gather information upon which to base reasonable hypotheses about the cause or causes of the patient's discomfort. Though the physician has at his disposal a number of methods of obtaining information, some based on observation, others based on instrumentation and laboratory procedures, the most important is the interview.

Interviewing is not, of course, unique to the doctor-patient relationship. It is the most common way of obtaining information to be used by professional persons in their relationships with clients, patients, and applicants. It also plays a role in many social relationships and brief business or professional encounters. Garrett writes:

> Everyone engages in interviewing. Sometimes he interviews; sometimes he is interviewed. The mother interviews the principal of the school in which she is thinking of entering her son. He, in turn, interviews the mother and the boy. Later the boy is interviewed by his prospective employer and, in turn, interviews the latter. Some people because of the nature of their work spend a good deal of time in interviewing. The attendant in an information booth devotes all his working hours to miniature interviews. Lawyers, doctors, nurses, newspapermen, policemen, ministers, counselors, creditmen, personnel managers, employers, all devote a considerable amount of time to talking with people, getting information from them, advising them, helping them.[1]

The physician is not the only health professional who uses interviewing to gather data upon which to base clinical decisions. With the broadening of the responsibilities of other members of the health care team, interviewing is now used in patient care by all of them. The hospital nurse conducts brief interviews which must be highly focused to collect data so that she can record the patient's physiological and psychological response to treatment. In outpatient health care, nurses may take initial histories, conduct screening interviews, and perform other interviewing tasks. In physicians' private offices, the nurse may be an informal psychotherapist. The social worker, member of a profession that has traditionally emphasized the development of skill in interviewing for data gathering and counseling, is assuming an increasingly important role in the health care team. Today, too, new health professionals who use interviewing are appearing. The physician's assistant, the nurse-practitioner, and the health aide are examples. Since the principles that we are about to discuss in this book apply to all interviewing in the care of patients, we will use the terms "doctor-patient relationship" and "clinician-patient relationship" interchangeably.

2 THE ART AND SCIENCE OF THE INTERVIEW

Kahn and Cannell define the interview as a specialized pattern of verbal interaction initiated for a specific purpose and focused on some specific content area, with consequent elimination of extraneous material.[2] This definition, while too broad,* clarifies an important aspect of the clinical interview: the interviewer not only must facilitate communication but at times must guide and even limit it. There are interviewing techniques, used mainly by some mental health professionals, that aim to facilitate communication almost exclusively, making little or no effort to limit it. While this may be necessary in conducting certain, though by no means all, types of psychotherapy, such an approach is inefficient and far too expensive to be generally appropriate in health care. It can be just as inefficient to ask too many highly specific questions early in an interview, as this may cut off communication or limit it prematurely.

In addition to communication skills, interviewing requires an attitude of openness as well as a basic curiosity—a desire to know

* Kahn and Cannell's definition could apply to any decision-making conference. It fails to clarify that in a clinical interview one person, the interviewer, has the major responsibility for the outcome. It should also be noted that during any interview the roles of interviewer and interviewee may reverse from time to time for brief or even long periods.

more about a person. The interviewer should have the capacity to transcend any cultural and social barriers between himself and the interviewee so that he can understand what the interviewee means by the words that he uses. And, of course, in medicine successful interviewing requires that the interviewer know enough about the patho-physiology of the illness and its clinical course as reflected in signs and symptoms to be able to evaluate the relevance of the information he obtains.

The mixture of art and science of clinical examination upon which the clinical decisions-making process rests is nowhere better described than in Feinstein's work *Clinical Judgement*.

> The art of clinical examination comes from attitudes and qualities that are neither obtained nor easily detected by scientific procedures: the clinician's awareness of people and human needs; his ability to temper the rational aspects of his work with a tolerant acceptance of the irrationalities of mankind; his perception of faith, hope, charity, love and other elements of human spirit and human emotion. These properties of care and of compassion, although sometimes dismissed as *merely* "bedside manner," are the fundamental and most important tools of any clinician. With them, he can often give healing or comfort where science fails or does not exist. Without them, his science is unsatisfactory, no matter how excellent.[3]

3 INTERVIEWING IN THE PROCESS OF PATIENT CARE

There is obviously an intimate relationship between interviewing and clinical decision-making. Every interview has the function of collecting information and ultimately leads to a decision. The decision may be simply to do nothing because more information is needed. Or it may be highly complex, involving the initiation of a course of therapy. The decision that stems from the interview might be that everything is going as well as could be expected and nothing need be changed. Clinical decision-making, is rarely a single isolated event. Except in those instances when the clinician-patient relationship begins and ends with a single encounter, as in an emergency room or crisis center, decision-making is continuous, both within a given period of illness and over longer periods of time that include episodes of illness and intervals of relatively good health. This is well known to family physicians and those other health professionals who are experienced in continuing medical care. Students and house officers are often far less aware of this and tend to think of a given interview as a complete, self-limiting transaction immediately after which a clinical decision must be made. The fact is that a tentative or preliminary decision might be made, but it is subject to revision with each subsequent interview. The corollary to this is that it is not necessary to gather all of the relevant data in one single interview. The astute clinician knows that he may begin his diagnostic studies with the first interview and that each subsequent interview will add increments of data that will increase the size of his "data bank" about his patient. Also, if the first interview is carried out with appropriate support, in such a way as to increase the patient's trust and confidence as well as his feeling of participation, the interviewer will probably obtain data with greater ease in subsequent encounters with the patient.

There is an often-quoted principle of scientific observation that entering any system or process, either as observer or participant, changes it. The interview has its effect, both on subsequent interviews and on the patient. Attitudes and expectations learned in each encounter have a significant influence on the patient's response to the doctor in the interviews that follow. This is especially true of the first interview that initiates the relationship and to a lesser extent, of the first in any episode of illness, in a continuing doctor-patient relationship. The clinician who biases his patient's account in the first interview will find that bias clouding his subsequent data and complicating the task of other clinicians who may take part in the patient's care.

In the chapters to follow, we will discuss the interview in data collection and recording, decision-making, and planning and instituting treatment. Interviewing as it pertains to every aspect of patient care is the central theme of this book.

REFERENCES

1. Garrett, A., *Interviewing: Its Principles and Methods*. New York: Family Service Association of America, 1942.
2. Kahn, R. L., and C. F. Cannell, *The Dynamics of Interviewing*. New York: John Wiley & Sons, Inc., 1957.
3. Feinstein, A. R., *Clinical Judgement*. Baltimore: The Williams and Wilkins Co., 1967.

2

THE NATURE OF MEDICAL INFORMATION

In Chapter 1 we stated that the function of the diagnostic interview is to collect information upon which to base clinical decisions, as well as to establish a helping relationship with the patient. This does not mean that data are collected first and decisions made later. As more data are gathered, the process of sorting and interpreting the available information goes on, and this includes the information about the patient collected by means other than interviewing, such as physical examination and laboratory studies.

1 BASIC CONCEPTS OF THE CHARACTER OF DATA

In the course of their education, most physicians have acquired some familiarity with the characteristics of "scientific" information. Not many are aware that they can use these same concepts in the examination of all the classes of information with which they work, including information derived by methods which are not classically scientific. It is our purpose here to review briefly some ideas that are fundamental to the understanding of all classes of information, then to show how these notions are also useful in dealing with the array of information which the clinician employs in the care of patients.

Measurement and Scales

The term "measurement" is most frequently applied to observations that are assigned numbers amenable to arithmetic manipulations. Many arithmetic operations apply to data measured on an interval scale, such as readings on a centigrade thermometer. The values on an interval scale are abitrary and ordered and meet the assumption that any two sets of numerically equidistant points on the scale represent equal differences in what is being measured. A ratio scale has the characteristics of an interval scale. In addition it has a true zero point, such as a measure of height or weight or a blood count. Ratio scales permit all arithmetic operations.

The human senses are the instruments utilized in many significant clinical observations; they employ scale values which reflect human judgments and are often expressed in the vocabulary of everyday language. These observations are sometimes systematized. They then may be described technically in terms of either nominal (classificatory) scales or ordinal scales. A nominal scale consists of a set of mutually exclusive subclasses. For example, individuals may be classified as either "sick" or "well." Greater precision may be introduced into a nominal scale by introducing additional, strictly defined subcategories. The subclass "sick" in the above example may be divided further into subclasses represented by diagnostic categories. If it is possible to rank order a set of subclasses with respect to the amount or degree of the property being measured, then that ordered set comprises an ordinal scale. The commonly used qualifiers "severe," "moderate," and "minimal" represent points on an ordinal scale. Heart murmurs are commonly graded in intensity with Roman numerals I through VI, which represent another example of an ordinal scale. The precision of an ordinal scale also may be increased by increasing the number of subclasses or recognizable differences, if this is possible. It is apparent that greater precision is possible with instruments which yield measurements on interval or ratio scales than by methods which yield measurements on nominal or ordinal scales. These subjectively determined scales are nevertheless useful as communication devices if they come to have some degree of common meaning to the people using them. They also have potential usefulness in applications of modern data processing techniques in medical practice.

Any datum has three primary dimensions: first, precision and accuracy, second, reliability and validity, and third, information content or value. The relationships among these three conceptual dimensions of a datum, relationships which determine its relevance in a given situation, are complex. Obviously these three dimensions are not entirely independent of each other in most real situations. It should be emphasized that the value of a datum is always related to its context—the total problem under consideration—and to the hierarchy of values imposed by the real world situation.

Precision and Accuracy

"Precision" may be defined as an expression of the degree of conformity which exists between an observation and that which has been observed. The precision of a measurement is closely related to the method by which the observation is made. For example, the diameter of a single plastic disc may be observed on three occasions with the following results: about an inch, an "eyeball" estimate; 1⅛ inches, the result of a rough measurement with a ruler; and 1.131 inches, the result of a measurement with a good micrometer. Each of these observations has a different degree of precision—low in the first case, where no instrument was used, high in the last instance, though still not absolute. With more sensitive methods, observations of even higher precision could be made if it were useful or necessary.

This brings us to the concept of *useful precision*. How precise need an observation be? The answer depends on the purpose for which the measurement was made. In general, increasing precision is increasingly costly. For every measurement, there is a degree of precision which justifies its cost. In the case of the plastic disc, the first observation is adequately precise if we wish to decide whether the disc is larger or smaller than a twenty-five-cent piece; the third level of observation may be inadequate if our problem is that of making a part for a precision machine. The penalty of excessive precision is excessive cost; the penalty of inadequate precision is a reduction in useful information. We will discuss this further in dealing with the notion of information content. The notion of useful precision is a part of ordinary judgment. Is it necessary to know that an event occurred yesterday, yesterday afternoon, yesterday about 3:00 p.m., or yesterday at 3:13 p.m.? The problem at hand will define the degree of precision with which the time of occurrence must be established.

"Accuracy" and "precision" are often used interchangeably, but they each have a specific meaning. "Precision" refers to the inherent sensitivity of a method of measurement. "Accuracy" reflects the calibration of that measurement against some recognized universal standard. For example, the measurements of a micrometer may be precise in that it can reliably detect differences of the order of 1×10^{-4} inches. Its accuracy will depend upon how closely it indicates 1.000 inches when it is used to measure a gauge block of this nominal dimension, a standard which in turn has been calibrated against a length standard of the U.S. Bureau of Standards.

The concepts of precision and accuracy can be useful in communication with patients. Communication is a process of information transfer. The precision with which you receive the patient's message may be worth consideration. Low precision, that is, a low degree of correspondence between what the patient said or meant and what you heard or translated into your own terms, results in a loss of information content.

Reliability and Validity

"Reliability of measurement" refers to the likelihood that the same results will be obtained if the same measuring procedures are reapplied under the same conditions. The likelihood that the same observer will obtain the same result if he reapplies a measurement is called "intra-observer reliability." The likelihood that different observers will obtain the same result is referred to as "inter-observer reliability."

Sometimes a population of events or subjects may be described with a single measure, for example, the mean weight of a group of newborns or the number of new cases of tuberculosis per 100,000 population. If we measure each individual in the population to be described, the reliability of the summary measure will depend on the reliability of the individual measurements. If, however, each individual in the population is not measured and only a sample is examined, then reliability refers to the probability that the same result would be obtained if we selected another sample of individuals from the same population under the same conditions. Under the same conditions, the reliability of the individual measurements may be high but that of the summary measure might be low. If the sample is selected by probability methods, the reliability of the summary measure may be calculated. The reliability of a summary measure then is dependent upon the reliability of the individual measurements, the size of the sample drawn, and the variability of the population with respect to the quality measured. A high precision measurement of a single member of a population will have low reliability in predicting the measurement of the next member when there is substantial variability. A relatively imprecise measurement, on the other hand, may be able to tell us with great reliability which are the largest and the smallest members of the group when variability is substantial.

The validity of an observation may be defined as a probability statement which expresses the likelihood that an observation one has made reflects the true status of the object or phenomenon observed. If the measurement is very strongly related to the object or event measured, then its degree of validity depends in large measure on the reliability, precision, and accuracy of the measurement. In the practice of medicine, we are generally more interested in the reliability of an observation than in its precision. For example, it is important to know that a patient's blood urea nitrogen (BUN) level is in the neighborhood of 40 mg./100 ml. and that upon repeated measurements values very close to this will be obtained. It is much less important to know that the value is precisely 40.13 mg./100 ml. on any one determination. A low precision method of measurement will result in low reliability of values which lie within the range of measurement error. Obviously, precision and reliability are related in connection with the value of an observation.

Information Content

In recent years, a method of dealing with information in quantitative terms called information theory has been developed to permit measurements of the likelihood that information will be garbled, lost, or distorted in communication systems. Some extensions of the concepts of information theory have been useful in biology and medicine.[1, 2] While it is neither feasible nor appropriate to develop these concepts fully here, it is important to recognize that information can be quantified and that there are ways of dealing with information content mathematically.

In general, we may say that information content of an observation is dependent upon the probability that it is related to one or more specific features of the situation being observed. Consider an observation that a very elderly patient is disoriented for time and place. A certain information content can be assigned to this observation on the basis of the high probability that the patient's brain function is abnormal. There is a further series of probabilities of an association of delirium with a range of organic diseases such as cerebral arteriosclerosis, uremia, cerebral neoplasm, and drug intoxication. On the other hand, the probabilities that the delirium is associated with a variety of other increasingly rare conditions are progressively lower. The information content of this observation is accordingly lower in these contexts. Observations which reflect essentially random events, those with low or zero probability of correlation with other features of the problem being studied, have low or zero information content with regard to the situation our problem is a part of.

A new discovery can be thought of as establishing a previously unrecognized probability that there is indeed an association of a given observation with a specific situation. This implies that the human mind has processes for recognizing potential information under conditions where the specific set of circumstances has not yet occurred often enough to permit a good estimate of the probabilities of a relationship.

We may summarize this brief discussion of the information content of medical observations by noting: information content must be considered in the context of the problem we are trying to solve, and information content is generally measured in terms of probabilities. The complex interdependence of precision, reliability, and information content of an observation should be apparent. Precision depends largely on how the observation was made. Reliability reflects the constancy or stability of the system being measured. Information content depends upon the probability that the measurement being made is correlated with some significant feature of the problem under study, such as the diagnosis or therapeutic response.

Two Clinical Considerations

The principle alluded to in Chapter 1, that observation alters that which is observed, is important in the assessment of the reliability of the information obtained in the interview. The interaction between patient and interviewer always alters, even if subtly, the patient's next recital of his story whether the next interview is conducted by the same or by a different observer. In general, it is likely that the first interview will yield the most uninfluenced version of the information, though subsequent interviews may give more information if conducted more skillfully. Preventing the introduction of bias into interviews is taken up in Chapter 4. I should be pointed out here that the first person to interview a patient has a responsibility to obtain the available data skillfully and accurately with minimum introduction of biases which can create difficulties in later interviews when the data may require extension or reevaluation.

Another useful concept is that of independence and interdependence of observations or measurements. Two observations are said to be independent when a change in the system determining one observation has no effect on the second. Because of the high degree of integration which characterizes whole body physiology and the unity of a patient's life situation, it is rare that multiple observations on a single individual are totally independent. For example, one would expect a high degree of independence between the blood hemoglobin concentration and the spinal fluid pressure. At the other extreme, the blood hemoglobin concentration and the hematocrit are very highly, but not completely, interdependent. In assessing the total amount of information we have about a problem, it is important to recognize that observations which are relatively independent are of the greatest value, while non-independent observations have their value in increasing the precision and reliability of the information. From the point of view of information theory, interdependent observations provide a type of redundancy of data.

The aim of the clinician is to develop a construct of the patient, his problems, and his situation on the basis of which a course of action is undertaken. This construct consists of data collected in the interview, by physical examination, and by laboratory procedures and the interrelationships among these data inferred by the clinician. Each datum contributes to this construct according to its information content. Each "signal" the clinician receives, in the terminology of information theory, contains a variety of "noises" which reduce or obscure the information content. These "noises" may represent invalid, unreliable, imprecise, or inaccurate information, or unrelated random events.

2 CLASSES OF MEDICAL INFORMATION

Information is gathered during the interview in two ways: by listening to what the patient says, guided by the interviewing behavior of the physician, and by observing the patient's behavior. The observations which are made about the way the patient walks, talks, holds himself, breathes, sits, and behaves toward the doctor are as important as the information gathered from the patient's words. From these two sources, observation of behavior and listening to the patient's account, four classes of information can be gathered. These are biological, psychological, social, and cultural.

Biological Information

Biological information generally reflects the pathological changes induced by the disease process as they influence the patient's functioning and subjective sensations. The aim of the physician is to observe these changes, to measure them where possible and to interpret them as pathological alterations of physiological processes. This information base is not equivalent to a diagnosis. Diagnosis proceeds from a second level of interpretation, in which a specific structural or functional abnormality is identified in relation to the observed changes. Diagnoses are in reality classifications of disease processes which provide a useful structural basis for knowledge about disease. A variety of systems of classification are employed. Classifications or diagnoses based upon etiology are most useful because the several categories tend to be mutually exclusive. Least useful are classifications based upon purely descriptive aspects of the pathology or clinical manifestations of a disease process.

Information can be obtained about the organic aspects of an illness in three forms: verbal, non-verbal, and data obtained through observation and physical or chemical measurement. Information in verbal form is the primary content of the interview. Non-verbal information is obtained through simultaneous and related observation and involves all the senses: vision, hearing, smell, taste, and touch, with or without instrumental extension. Both verbal and non-verbal data may be recorded in words with varying degrees of precision, and in some cases may be expressed in quantitative terms. Non-verbal data are also derived through procedures which make measurements beyond primary sensory perceptions. They usually are obtained and recorded in numerical form. Data expressed in numbers are ordinarily of high precision when compared with the non-denumerable data obtained in the interview. They also appear to be more "objective." But the verbal and non-verbal interview data, if skilfully collected, will be high in information content and of prime importance in problem-solving.

Verbal data arise from the patient's own description of his discomfort, his behavior, and the pathophysiological changes he has observed which have led him to consult a physician. The type of onset and pattern of pain, other discomfort or limitation of function, the frightening manifestations of unexpected bleeding or discharges, the alterations in appearance such as change in skin color, all can be put together to give a picture of the patient's biological status. Sometimes, a classic picture drawn by the patient of the onset, nature, and precipitants of his pain can be interpreted as a pathophysiological diagnosis with great accuracy, as in the case of clear-cut angina pectoris. In other instances, biological information gained in the interview makes it possible to restrict the number of diagnostic laboratory procedures needed to establish a diagnosis to a very few. But a diagnosis alone is insufficient in most instances to permit adequate and effective treatment; knowledge of the patient and his life situation are usually of great importance. More than diagnosis is necessary for a supportive ongoing relationship with the patient that is essential to effective health care.

Psychological Information

Psychological factors play a role in many illnesses. Sometimes the underlying cause of an illness has more to do with the patient's psychological state than with his physical state. Sometimes the psychological reaction to illness may overshadow the physical illness. The patient's psychological reaction to the clinician may play an important role in the interview as well as in treatment. The relevant information about psychological status includes the patient's mood, his response to the clinician, his attitude toward himself and others around him, the way he communicates and expresses himself, his perceptions, his thinking processes, and his intelligence.

The patient's psychological status is usually adduced both from his story and from his behavior. The subjective verbal account is referred to as the *content* of the interview. The object in eliciting this content is to permit the patient the opportunity for self-reporting. In other words, the patient is encouraged to relate verbally all those inner experiences of which he is aware and which motivate him to seek health care. But what is verbally communicated is only part of the picture. Verbal self-reporting may be limited by embarrassment, hostility, fear, lack of knowledge, and so forth. Thus, no matter how rich and detailed the patient's verbal account may be, it is not enough. The other significant source of information is the patient's behavior. The manner in which the patient behaves as he interacts with the doctor is the *process* of the interview. The patient usually demonstrates objective (i.e. behavioral) signs of the various difficulties that he experiences. These include signs of internal discomfort, such as the manifestations of tension, anxiety, and depression. The patient's speech, by its rhythm, intonations, and silences, may point to significant problem areas. The interview is an interpersonal situation and, therefore, provides important information concerning the characteristic behavioral style of the patient as he relates to another individual. Signs of interpersonal difficulties, such as withdrawal, dependency, attempts to dominate or be dominated, and the manipulation of others, can be obtained from studying interview behavior. Thus, the range of information available to the clinician includes the subjective content of the patient's story and the more objective observations of behavior made during the process of the interview.[3]

Content and process give the information that is sometimes referred to as the mental status. As will be discussed in Chapters 4 and 5, one should, in recording mental status, describe the patient's attitude and behavior, his way of relating to the interviewer, his mood and its appropriateness to his situation, and his thinking. Under the category of thinking are included his concerns, preoccupations, trends of thought, ability to reason and to think logically, memory, and the presence or absence of obsessions, delusions, and hallucinations.

A useful, if crude, assessment of the patient's intelligence can be made during a clinical interview. Intelligence is not an absolute measure; nor is the I.Q. a valid measure of all patients' intellectual functioning. Intelligence test results are influenced by emotional, personality, and social-cultural factors. What is referred to as intelligence and what we try to measure includes the ability to understand and deal effectively with abstract ideas and symbols, the ability to learn, and the ability to act reasonably in new situations. In a clinical interview we are able to assess, in a rough way, whether or not the patient has the intelligence to comprehend his own situation, give reasonably accurate information about himself, and cooperate in his own treatment.

Failure on the part of the clinician to make himself understood or to understand a patient may have little or nothing to do with the patient's intelligence, however. People from some subcultures and from lower socio-economic groups and those who have modest formal education may be quite intelligent but speak a different sort of language than the interviewer does. Social distance between clinician and interviewer may lead to a mistakenly low evaluation of the patient's intelligence.

Social Information

Socio-economic status is an important variable in the type of illness a patient might have. It also influences the way a patient perceives symptoms and his decision as to whether they warrant his seeking health care. Socio-economic status is in addition a determinant of the physical and environmental factors that might play a role in the production as well as the treatment of illness. Among the disorders that have been correlated with socio-economic status are hypertension, peptic ulcers, breast cancer, and coronary artery disease.[4] It is important then to gather information that will make it possible to assess the patient's socio-economic status. In studying socio-economic stratification of a small northeastern city, Hollingshead[5] concluded that in assigning families to a class position, the most consideration was given to where a family lived, the way it made its living, its tastes, its cultural orientation, and the way it spent its leisure time. The patient's address, or neighborhood, correlates with socio-economic status with rather high accuracy. The educational level of the head of the household, whether or not that person is the patient, is a good index to social class. Occupation was ranked by Hollingshead in the following order: first, executives and proprietors of large concerns, and major professionals; second, managers and proprietors of medium-size businesses, and lesser professionals; third, administrative personnel of large concerns, owners of small independent businesses, and semi-professionals; fourth, owners of very small businesses, clerical and sales workers, and technicians; fifth, skilled workers; sixth, semi-skilled workers; and seventh, unskilled workers.

Social mobility is another factor that can be correlated with certain disorders. Social mobility may be vertical, that is, an individual may move to a higher or to a lower social class, or it may be horizontal, such as might occur in divorce and remarriage or in moving from one job to another, similar job. A mobile individual is likely to be exposed to social stress arising form new relationships and responsibilities and it is then necessary to make a series of personal adjustments. There is some evidence that social movement may create difficulties of such magnitude that they are the equivalent of a life crisis. Neurosis, peptic ulcer, and proneness to infectious disease have been connected with upward mobility.[6] Parker and Kleiner present evidence that in Negroes both upward and downward social mobility correlate with significantly higher rates of mental illness than social stability does.[7]

Koos[8] has shown that the assessment of the significance of common symptoms varies with socio-economic status. He presented people living in a small town with a list of seventeen easily recognizable symptoms and asked which of them should be called to the attention of the doctor. The responses indicate not only the symptoms for which a doctor might be consulted but also those which are likely to be reported spontaneously during a clinical interview.

While 100 per cent of those in the community's business and

professional class felt that blood in the urine should be reported and 98 per cent felt that blood in the stool should be reported, only 69 per cent of the lowest class stated that blood in the urine should be reported, while 60 per cent said they would report blood in the stool. Only 19 per cent of the lowest class considered persistent backache, persistent joint and muscle pains, and chronic fatigue to be symptoms appropriate to report to a physician. Fifty-three per cent of the upper class stated they would report persistent backache and 80 per cent of the upper class would report the symptoms of persistent joint and muscle pain and of chronic fatigue. Upper- and middle-class people indicated that loss of appetite was a medical problem. A much smaller percentage of poor people thought so. More than three-fourths of the upper-class people thought that fifteen of the seventeen symptoms presented were medical problems; no symptom of the seventeen was considered to be a reason to go to the doctor by as many as three-fourths of the persons in the lowest class. The blue-collar workers tended to fall somewhere between the high number of upper-class people and the low number of lower-class people who viewed each symptom as medically significant.

The structure of the patient's family is important social information. Illness, response to illness, and the ease or difficulty of carrying out treatment all relate in varying ways to the individual's position in a family. The major role of the family, other than child-rearing, is the provision of emotional support to its members. The number of divorces, conflicted marriages, and troubled parent-child relationships encountered in our society testify eloquently to the fragility of the family in the face of its responsibilities. It is apparent that illness throws a heavy additional burden on the family, which may already have reached its point of maximum tolerance of economic and emotional stress. A family member who has become ill often cannot continue to carry out his family role. The loss of economic support when a husband and father becomes ill and the loss of love and emotional support when a wife and mother becomes ill will have an upsetting effect on the entire family, undermining a precariously balanced emotional or financial security—often both. Often the patient's behavior is affected as much by reactions to his illness from overburdened and overstressed family members as by any other aspect of his illness.

Illness can be used as a way out by a wife and mother who can no longer tolerate the emotional burdens on her. The father who becomes unemployed or unemployable may find sickness an acceptable justification for failing to play the socially approved, breadwinner role or failing to exercise his authority in the family. For the child, illness may provide an escape from increasingly exacting requirements that he behave like a grown-up, and it can be a way of securing more maternal love when this seems to be spread too thinly within the family. Illness in the child may rob the husband of some much-needed support from his wife, with consequent ill effects on him and a change in his response to both his wife and the sick child.

To be maximally useful in making decisions and planning patient care, a medical interview clearly should gather information about the family and information from the family. The interactional process within the family may determine who is sick, and why he is. Later in this book, we will discuss the interview of the family in greater detail.

An important piece of social information is the patient's occupation. Many industrial diseases are associated with specific occupations, such as coal mining, factory work with chemicals, and farm work with exposure to pesticides. It is useful to have exact information about the patient's specific job and, where appropriate, his exposures and their duration.

Cultural Information

Society may be viewed as a system of social relationships. Culture is defined as the content of these relationships. In other words, the way of life of an ethnic group or society, its language, attitudes, skills, value systems, and shared ethical judgments, make up its culture.[6] The ethnic group to which the patient belongs may be very important in assessing the patient's problems and in planning treatment.

Cultural factors will influence what a patient regards or reports as illness, as well as the way he reports it. This is highlighted by some studies of very divergent cultures. For example, the Kuba of Sumatra, who carry on a difficult way of life in the primeval forest, have a high incidence of injuries to the skin and skin diseases. The person with a skin disease is not considered a sick man among the Kuba.[9] A Kuba consulting a physician would thus be unlikely to report a skin lesion. Bloom, in his discussion of the cultural differences in defining illness, describes a 1911 report of a Rockefeller Commission on Hookworm which found a whole region in North Africa where hookworm was regarded as a normal condition and public health measures to correct it were violently opposed.[10]

Some interesting cultural differences in the way pain is described have been reported. Navajo language, for example, does not include words to indicate the various forms of pain which the dominant white culture recognizes. Navajos consequently have difficulty telling a doctor whether the pain is sharp, dull, cutting, and so on.[11] Zborowski studied the response to pain in patients of Old American, Jewish, Irish, and Italian origin.[12] The Jewish and Italian patients were described as emphasizing or "playing up" their perception of pain, describing all pain as "very severe." Old American and Irish tended to de-emphasize or "play down" pain and were more apt to differentiate between slight, severe, and very severe pain. Old Americans tended to report pain unemotionally. The Irish offered "vague and confused" information. The Jewish patients could describe pain with great precision but could not differentiate degree. The Old Americans could describe pain precisely as well as differentiate degree. It was difficult to determine the nature, location, and duration of the pain described by Irish and Italian patients. Motor responses to pain, such as body movements, gestures, twisting, and jumping were common in Jewish and Italian patients, non-expressive behavior most common in the Old Americans and Irish. Jewish patients tended to consult their physicians promptly after becoming aware of pain or discomfort, while Old Americans and, to a lesser extent, Irish patients tended to delay consultation with a physician. Old Americans and Irish had the greatest confidence in the doctor's skill, while Jewish patients had the least, tending to check up on doctors, to shop around, and to insist on explanations of the meaning and significance of their pain.

Failure to appreciate the characteristic responses to symptoms can lead to misdiagnosis, so that in a given ethnic group "organic" conditions can be mistakenly diagnosed as "psychiatric" disorders. An example of this was described by Zola who studied lower-class Italians, Irish, and Anglo-Saxons seeking aid at the medical, eye, and ear-nose-and-throat clinics of a large urban hospital. He found that proportionately more Italian patients were labeled "psychiatric problems" by their physicians, despite a lack of evidence that psycho-social problems were more frequent among them.[13, 14] In urban metropolitan regions there may be many subcultures identifiable as ethnic groups. In rural areas there may be fewer subcultures and less social stratification. In today's highly mobile society, people tend to migrate frequently, so that it is important to identify regional subcultures, such as Deep South, border southern states, Texas, California, and New England. There are subcultures that are both regional and ethnic (Spanish-Americans from New Mexico, Southwest American Indians, North Carolina American Indians, etc.).

Other subcultures are defined by membership in a religious group, such as Southern Baptist, Seventh Day Adventist, and Jehovah's Witnesses. The latter two have values and customs of specific medical significance. Most Seventh Day Adventists are vegetarian and do not drink alcoholic beverages or smoke. Jehovah's Witnesses will not permit a blood transfusion.

There are also generational subcultures. Teenagers share a large number of values and attitudes that differ from those of middle-age people, for example. They have their own way of life as exemplified in their langauge, dress, and social habits.

Of course, this discussion is not meant to imply that all members of a subculture share all of the same values, attitudes, and customs. Individual variations are influenced by such factors as geographic mobility and exposure to other cultures, degree of assimilation, and amount of education.

The interviewer should not attempt to predict a patient's behavior from knowledge of his social class or ethnicity. No individual can be counted on to behave according to sociological descriptions of his group. Before drawing conclusions from a patient's surname, one should also take into consideration the number of generations the family has resided in the United States, the patient's marital status, level of education, occupation, and the presence or absence of an accent, characteristic gestures, or other signs of subcultural identity. Ethnic and other subcultural influences on a patient should be assessed by the interviewer through observation, with attention to the patient's speech and manner as well as by obtaining specific social historical data.

Sources of Information

While the most important single source of information (except in very severely ill or comatose patients) is the patient himself, there are other significant sources for the data needed to arrive at an accurate diagnosis and to plan treatment. Perhaps the best collateral source is the patient's family. In the case of children, the family is, of course, an indispensible source of information. There are instances when the interview is limited to the patient; others in which the family is also seen; and still others in which the family, or part of it, is interviewed as a group. This will be discussed further in Chapter 8.

Other sources of information that may be employed include physicians previously consulted, the social worker, the visiting nurse in the instance of home care, previous medical records, and in rare instances the employer, personnel department of a large company, and school authorities.

REFERENCES

1. Goldman, Stanford, *Information Theory*. New York: Prentice-Hall, 1953.
2. Yockey, H. P., R. L. Platzman, and H. Quastler, *Information Theory in Biology*. New York: Pergamon Press, 1956.
3. Enelow, A. J., and M. Wexler, *Psychiatry in the Practice of Medicine*. New York: Oxford University Press, 1966, p. 38.
4. Graham, S., "Social Factors in Relation to Chronic Illness," in H. E. Freeman, S. Levine, and L. F. Reeder (eds.), *Handbook of Medical Sociology*. Englewood Cliffs, N.J.: Prentice-Hall, 1963, pp. 65-98.
5. Hollingshead, A. B., and F. C. Redlich, *Social Class and Mental Illness*. New York: John Wiley & Sons. Science Editions (paper), 1964.
6. Susser, M. W., and W. Watson, *Sociology in Medicine*. London: Oxford University Press, 1971.
7. Parker, S., and R. J. Kleiner, *Mental Illness in the Urban Negro Community*. New York: The Free Press, 1966.
8. Koos, E. L., *The Health of Regionville*. New York: Hafner, 1967 (reprinted).
9. Sigerist, H. E. Cited in: S. W. Bloom, *The Doctor and His Patient*. New York: The Free Press, 1965 (paper), p. 99.
10. Bloom, S. W., *The Doctor and His Patient*. New York: The Free Press, 1965 (paper).
11. King, S. H., *Perceptions of Illness and Medical Practice*. New York: Russell Sage Foundation, 1962, p. 67.
12. Zborowski, M., *People in Pain*. San Francisco: Jossey-Bass, 1969.
13. Zola, I. K., "Problems of Communications, Diagnosis, and Patient Care: The Interplay of Patient, Physician and Clinic Organization," *Journal of Medical Education*, 38:829, 1963.
14. Zola, I. K., "Culture and Symptoms: An Analysis of Patients' Presenting Complaints," *American Sociological Review*, 31:615, 1966.

3

BASIC INTERVIEWING

Allen J. Enelow, M.D., and
Leta McKinney Adler, Ph.D.

1 THE CLINICIAN-PATIENT RELATIONSHIP

What we would term an effective clinician-patient relationship is ideally characterized by trust and confidence in the clinician; a feeling of relative autonomy and appropriate participation on the part of the patient; continuity of the relationship with flexibility in its nature and depth; and reasonable expectations on the part of both doctor and patient.

Trust and Confidence

Illnesses that cause people to seek help are very often accompanied by anxiety, a feeling of helplessness, and disturbances of the relationships between the patient and others around him. Often, too, illness leads to a disruption of family functioning and to loss or threatened loss of income. Therefore, the patient comes to the physician with a characteristic mixture of hope and fear. He hopes that the physician will be able to discover the cause of his discomfort and take appropriate steps to set things right. At the same time, he fears that the physician may not be able to help him and, in some instances, that help is not possible. These fears may be compounded by apprehension over the cost of care, or the possibility of painful, disabling, or disfiguring treatment procedures.

Initial trust in the physician's professional skill is usually created by the degree of confidence the physician communicates by his manner and by such things as diplomas, certificates, and office atmosphere. It is another thing, however, to have a feeling of personal trust and confidence in the physician. Trust and confidence are built when the physician provides support and when he respects the patient's autonomy. They are also created when the physician (or other clinician) maintains the reserve that defines him as a professional person whose aim is to help, and who seeks no reward from the relationship beyond those given to the professional person for being successful in his work. Of course, previous successful treatment of the patient or his family or friends also provides a basis for trust.

Autonomy and Participation

Three types of doctor-patient relationship have been described by Szasz and Hollender: activity-passivity, guidance-cooperation, and mutual participation.[1] The major variables in the three relationships are the degree of participation and feeling of autonomy on the part of the patient.

In the activity-passivity relationship, the physician uses all of the authority inherent in his status, and the patient feels no autonomy, tries hard to please the physician, and does not actively participate in his treatment. While usually required in the management of emergencies, it is the poorest type of relationship for diagnostic interviewing and data-gathering, as well as for much treatment.

In the guidance-cooperation type of doctor-patient relationship, the physician still exercises much authority and the patient is obedient, but the patient has a greater feeling of autonomy and participates somewhat more actively in the relationship. This is more appropriate than the activity-passivity model for a diagnostic interview. But a guidance-cooperation relationship does not encourage emergence of the widest possible range of relevant information. The desire to please the physician still may cause the patient to restrict information to what he perceives is wanted, as well as to bias the information he gives in a direction that seems to be desired by the interviewer. Alertness and great skill in phrasing questions on the part of the interviewer are necessary in order to overcome this tendency. Later in the interview, during the detailed inquiry commonly called the review of systems, a guidance-cooperation relationship is appropriate.

The mutual participation relationship is the most desirable for the diagnostic interview, as it is for the management of chronic illness. Here the patient feels some responsibility for a successful outcome, which involves both active participation and a feeling of relatively great personal autonomy, that is to say, responsibility for his own behavior. This is created by appropriate moderation of the physician's use of his authority, a theme that will recur throughout this chapter. In such a relationship, the widest range of relevant diagnostic information tends to emerge and the most successful outcome of treatment is likely to occur. While it is true that some dependence on the physician is useful, especially in acute and frightening illness, it is generally not useful to foster the patient's feeling of dependence. Dependence can reach a point where it interferes with treatment and prolongs the relationship. The best clinician-patient relationships encourage the patient to take increasing responsibility for himself, at a time and rate consistent with good treatment.

Continuity and Flexibility

While the clinician-patient relationship ideally has continuity, it is characteristically flexible in both nature and depth. There are times when the relationship is intense and involves frequent contacts and detailed explorations of the patient's physical and personal life. At other times, the relationship is casual and occasional, perhaps consisting of an annual checkup or help for a minor and limited disorder, such as a simple laceration or sprain. The nature of the relationship may vary from the careful exploration of unexplained severe and acute symptoms to counseling, and from routine procedures such as inoculations or superficial physical examinations to intensely emotional encounters during times of stress or crisis in the patient's life. In the most successful clinician-patient relationships a data bank is built through repeated encounters. New information is added as each new problem is explored and its solution sought. The ability to establish this kind of relationship is primarily a function of the emotional and supportive aspects of the interview.

Reasonable Expectations

The patient's expectations from the doctor-patient relationship, and therefore from the interview, are very much influenced by the pain and fear he is experiencing when he consults the doctor. The patient expects to have the source of his disorder found and corrected. He also expects some degree of comforting or care from the physician and some reassurance. His view of a successful outcome of his treatment is that it produce a positive feeling of well-being, not just the absence of pain or discomfort. The fact that this outcome is not always possible is never easily accepted by patients, except for those who are "professional patients," that is, those who have learned to obtain gratification from the sick role. It is important that the physician deal realistically with the patient's expressed and unexpressed expectations from him and from their relationship. Open and frank discussions about prognosis are usually helpful; tact and an understanding of appropriate timing are necessary.

2 THE INTERVIEW MODEL

What kind of interview is most likely to produce a relationship characterized by trust and confidence, an appropriate degree of autonomy and participation, flexibility in its nature and depth, and reasonable expectations on the part of the patient? It is our view that an open-ended interviewing style is most likely to produce the desired type of clinical relationship and to be both effective and efficient in the task of data collection.

Before describing this open-ended model, let us examine two alternative approaches to interviewing. Our observations of physicians in postgraduate courses and of house officers in university hospital clinics led us to conclude that the average medical interviewer is likely to seek information in the most direct manner possible—by asking a great many questions. This style of interviewing might be called directive-interrogative. It is often referred to as history-taking. The physician has a long "list" of items in mind about which he wishes to have information. Each bit of information given to him by the patient is followed by several specific questions elucidating details. In a number of observed situations, certain consistent effects of this interview style were noted. The patient has a tendency to become quite passive. Often the patient makes some early efforts to bring in personal concerns, then ceases the efforts and limits his communication to supplying the information that is being sought. When the interviewer and the patient come from different cultures or different social classes, the patient may struggle to understand the interviewer with limited success. The interviewer often responds with increasingly specific questions (and sometimes with irritability). The relationship has rarely deepened by the conclusion of the interview. Important diagnostic clues, particularly in the psychological and social areas, may not be picked up.

In the mental health care disciplines, by contrast, one is likely to find very little emphasis on fact-finding through an inquisitory technique and a much greater emphasis on the development of rapport. Much attention is paid to the empathic responses of the interviewer and to the facilitation of communication, and correspondingly less attention to data collection. Facts are not actively sought; they are permitted to emerge. This is especially true of the psychiatric interview that will lead to psychotherapy and of the social worker's casework interview.[2]

The open-ended interview to be described here is a derivative of the interview styles that have emerged in the mental health professions. It has been modified to fit the medical or health care setting. It combines the goals of the fact-finding type of interview with the concern for rapport and the emphasis on emergence of information, rather than the extraction of facts, that characterize the interviewing style of most mental health professionals. The description of the characteristics of the open-ended interview and the most likely responses of patients to the interview behaviors of the physician are based on five years of research in interviewing, using an interaction analysis scale developed by Adler and Enelow.[3, 4, 5] The guiding principle of the open-ended interview is that the clinician should exert the least amount of authority necessary to obtain the information he is seeking within the time allotted for the interview.

There are four general characteristics of this style of interviewing. First, the interview should be carried out in an atmosphere that encourages spontaneous behavior on the part of the patient. Second, the interviewer's behavior should encourage communication. Third, the interviewer should give attention to the patient's non-verbal behavior as well as his story. Fourth, the interviewer's specific information-seeking actions should be those that exercise the least control first, and the highest degree of control as late in the interview as possible.[6]

The Atmosphere of the Interview

An atmosphere that encourages spontaneous behavior has both physical and emotional attributes. Comfort and privacy should be provided whenever possible. The interviewer should arrange for the fewest possible interruptions.

The interviewer's behavior should encourage communication.

The interviewer should communicate by his manner that the patient can respond freely and discuss whatever he wishes. As a rule of thumb, the fewer the clinician's utterances to keep the patient talking, the better. This is especially true in the earlier part of the interview.

The interviewer should give attention to the patient's non-verbal behavior as well as his story.

Non-verbal communication is often more indicative of a patient's inner state than his verbal account. Information not contained in words may be clearly expressed in behavior, manner, and appearance. An important way of facilitating the patient's spontaneous account is to call his attention to the observed behavior.

The interviewer should move through a cycle of information-seeking behavior that begins with low use of authority and proceeds to progressively greater use of authority.

The interview is best opened with a broad open-ended question such as "What kind of difficulties are you having?" As the patient answers, the interviewer should encourage spontaneous elaboration on his account through facilitating remarks and gestures. If the interviewer observes that that patient is encountering difficulty in describing his problems or discomfort, or finds it difficult to understand his account, he should point it out to the patient. If there is incongruity between the patient's behavior and his account, the patient's attention should be drawn to the observed behavior. Lastly, if these methods have not yielded specific items of needed information, or at that point in the interview where specific details are needed to fill in the story, the interviewer should use direct questions.

The principle is this: spontaneous reporting tends to produce the broadest range of information, most of which is likely to be relevant. When verbal communication ceases, non-verbal communication continues. Pointing out the non-verbal behavior tends to encourage the verbal expression of the inner experience. For example, a patient who is told that he has a worried and pained look may then describe his chronic low-grade neck stiffness and headache. Feelings, such as sadness or fear, may be first expressed after the non-verbal (behavioral) evidence has been brought to his attention. If this does not succeed, questioning may be necessary. If the patient can express himself well, very few questions may be necessary. A very important reason for limiting the interviewer's control over the patient's communication is to minimize bias in the information offered. The wording, timing, and sequence of questions, as well as non-verbal behavior accompanying them, all may provide cues that influence the patient's replies.

3 BASIC INTERVIEWING TECHNIQUES

Opening the Interview

The open-ended question, such as "What kind of troubles have you been having?" says to the patient, "I am interested in anything you may feel is important enough to you to tell me." In return interviews, an appropriate variant might be, "How have you been getting along?" Interviewers who do not use the open-ended question frequently close off whole veins of important information since they do not give the patient permission to develop areas not covered by the interviewer. Yet some patients, especially children and adolescents but also adults, are unable to respond to an open-ended question with a detailed account. In such a case the interviewer may be tempted to begin direct questioning at once. If the sole reply to "What kind of troubles have you been having?" is "Well, I've been having a lot of headaches," followed by silence, the clinician may fall into the trap of asking a series of questions like "How long have you had them?", "How long do they last?", "Where does the pain seem to be?", "What relieves them?", and so on. Each specific question the doctor asks will increase the probability that the patient will give the exact information requested and lapse into silence awaiting the next question.

Before embarking on a line of direct specific questioning the interviewer should try less controlling actions. These are silence, facilitation, and, if appropriate, confrontation.

Silence

The least controlling thing an interviewer can do is to be silent and "give the patient the floor." If the patient falls silent, the interviewer should consider being silent himself for at least a brief time. Ordinarily the patient will soon feel free to resume his account. That the clinician is not speaking does not mean that he is not communicating. His facial expression, posture, and movements all tell the patient something about the interviewer's response to his account and to him as a person. An attentive facial expression and posture tell the patient non-verbally that he has an interested listener. On the other hand, standing over a bed patient suggests that you will not remain long enough for him to tell you very much. It is a good idea to look at the patient but not stare continuously into the patient's eyes. Looking distracted, fidgeting, slumping in an attitude of fatigue, looking away from the patient, and examining the chart all indicate that the interviewer's attention is not fully focused on the patient. This non-verbal message will inhibit the patient considerably.

Thus while the patient is communicating freely about important matters, the doctor's behavior of choice is an interested, attentive, and relaxed silence. Whether to remain silent or to speak when the patient falls silent is a choice which requires the skill that comes with experience. During an interview silences of only a few seconds often seem interminably long. Silence is frequently quite uncomfortable for the inexperienced interviewer. The busy practitioner is also likely to tolerate silences poorly because of his schedule consciousness. A common response of both beginner and busy practitioner is to search for a question or a remark to keep the conversation going. But one can learn to tolerate silences through practice. This is a worthwhile exercise as there are times when it is very useful to the interview for the clinician to maintain his silence after the patient has stopped speaking.

One of these times is when the patient has stopped speaking in order to clarify his thoughts, to recollect facts, or to find a way of adequately expressing something. The patient may explain such silences with remarks like, "Let me think a minute," or "How can I say that better?" This kind of thoughtful silence is rarely accompanied by signs of increased tension. The perceptive interviewer can usually recognize this situation and wait for the patient to continue. An interruption may make it more difficult for the patient to express himself clearly.

Another situation requiring a decision whether to remain silent or to initiate some action occurs when the patient appears to have said all he wants to say and has come to a natural pause. The pause may be signaled by a remark and by the patient's demeanor indicating that he has finished and is waiting to hear from you. The best choice at this juncture depends on a number of circumstances.

First, the clinician should consider how often these pauses have been occurring and how lengthy and complete the patient's narrative has been. If the patient has been limiting his remarks to a few phrases or sentences, then waiting for you to take the initiative again, you may have been interrogating him. If you have been asking a great many direct questions, continuing after brief replies, the patient will assume that brief replies in response to your questions are what you wish and expect. If, upon reflection, you feel you have placed yourself in such a situation, a pause on your part may encourage the patient to go on. If the patient continues to remain silent, it may be helpful to try a comment or facilitation with a relatively low level of control.

If, after reflecting on the course of the interview, you realize that you have been working hard to help the patient tell his story on his own, and you sense that the patient is "holding back" and that his non-verbal behavior reflects tension or discomfort, your silence is again likely to be appropriate: in the silence which follows, the patient's discomfort may well increase, and he may then tell you on his own what is bothering him and give you an opportunity to deal with it. This could be something in the immediate environment, such as telephone interruptions, the intrusion of office personnel, or a feeling that you are uninterested. On the other hand, it may be reticence, shame, or embarrassment about telling important parts of his story. The difficulty in communication which has developed may also be due to the patient's discomfort in speaking freely to someone of different sex, age, class, race, or ethnic background. The patient may fear the possible diagnosis and react to this anxiety by failing to communicate freely in order to "ward off" the knowledge that he has the disease he dreads. Or his discomfort may be related to important events or circumstances in his personal life that you need to know about in order to manage the patient's treatment successfully. Whatever the reason for his evasiveness and discomfort, a pause will allow his discomfort to become clearly evident to both of you. If he does not speak about it spontaneously, you are ready to point out the difficulties in communicating which you have been observing. A confrontation in this situation will frequently result in a discussion of the difficulty the patient is encountering. This will usually permit the interview to proceed smoothly.

The situation in which a patient has been communicating freely but shows increasing difficulty with a particular topic and halts the account is another instance of silence best handled by remaining silent. In the ensuing pause, the emotional basis for the failure of communication may become apparent, and the clinician can then proceed with a confrontation leading to a discussion of the difficulty.

There is one time when it is mandatory for the clinician to remain silent. This is when the patient has stopped speaking because he is overwhelmed, or about to be overwhelmed, by emotion. Sometimes one may forestall or attenuate an expression of strong emotion, most frequently weeping, by prematurely saying something to the patient, thereby failing to reduce the patient's tension. There are several reasons for remaining silent until the patient has expressed strong emotion and brought his feelings under control. Foremost is that open expression of feelings is almost always therapeutic for a patient. In addition, it is likely that a patient will be able to express himself more adequately after a release of emotion. He may well be able to speak of things which he could not bring himself to discuss before. If, on the other hand, the patient decides to control himself and withhold his feelings, he has the opportunity to do so. He makes the choice himself; it is not forced on him.

The extent to which the patient is helped and the interview is facilitated by permitting a display of feeling depends very much on what the doctor says and does after it has subsided. A supportive response is almost always helpful. This will be taken up in a later part of this chapter.

In some cases it will not be appropriate for you to remain silent when a patient pauses. If an overly talkative patient who has been dominating the interview and preventing the efficient gathering of diagnostic information stops talking, for example, you might take the opportunity to obtain some of the information you need. Another time that you would not necessarily remain silent at the patient's pause would be when you felt a need for clarification of what the patient had been saying. There are several ways you might choose to proceed and they will be described later.

In the early part of an interview, silence may allow the patient to go on to a new topic. If the patient shows signs of increasing tension as a silence develops, one can acknowledge what was just said, ask a broad question concerning this or other problems the patient may have, or comment on the patient's discomfort. Near the close of the interview, when the interviewer feels he has a generally complete account of the patient's situation, he may not pause but instead immediately move to obtain some specific information with questions.

There are a few "don'ts" with regard to the use of silence on the part of interviewer. Most individuals in our society are made uncomfortable by long silences in ordinary conversation. A doctor who overuses silence may be perceived by the patient as cold or distant. Certain individuals, particularly adolescents, do not tolerate silence well. When the interviewer perceives that his silence produces discomfort in his patient to the point of reducing further communication, he should become more active.

Facilitation

Encouraging communication by manner, gesture, or words that do not specify the kind of information sought is called facilitation. It represents a greater use of authority than silence but still exerts a low degree of control. Since a completely impassive silence on the part of the interviewer is relatively uncommon, silence and facilitation tend to go hand in hand. An interested, attentive manner is, of course, facilitating. Any change of facial expression or posture displaying greater interest or attention is a facilitation. A common mode of facilitation is the nod of the head, conveying, "I'm listening," "I understand what you're saying," or "Go on." This message is encouraging to the patient but can be overused. Inexperienced interviewers frequently relieve their own tension during the interview with what might be called the "head-nodding syndrome." The clinician should also take pains not to nod his head for facilitating purposes when the patient has been expressing a strong opinion. In such instances, his action may be mistaken for approval or agreement.

A similar message is conveyed to the patient with an occasional "mmm-mmm" or by postural shifts toward the patient or into a position of greater alertness. The doctor may also interject short words or phrases such as "Yes" or "I see" without interrupting the flow of the patient's narrative.

Another type of message that is facilitating is the action that conveys "I don't understand." This may be non-verbal, such as a puzzled look, or a verbal statement of confusion on the order of "I don't follow you" or "I'm sorry, but I don't understand."

When a patient has stopped or appears to be about to stop discussing a topic and the interviewer wants more information, he also may encourage the patient to continue by repeating his last few words. This may be done with the inflection of a question or merely as a repetition. For example, either "the last few days" or "the last few days?" will invite the patient to continue. Another verbal facilitation is a brief summary of what the patient has been saying. This indicates that you have understood him and are interested in further information. A brief summarizing remark will usually encourage the patient to continue, without explicitly directing him to do so or specifying what subject he should discuss.

Facilitation can also be used to return the patient to a topic previously introduced. This is done by referring back to a phrase previously used by the patient which indicates the matter of interest to the clinician. For example, in the course of describing her child's respiratory complaints, a mother may mention that her child has had fever and then go on without elaborating. After she has completed her description, the physician can then say, "You say Johnny has had some fever?"

Facilitation, then, evokes communication by suggesting to the patient that the doctor is interested in what the patient is saying and is encouraging him to continue. It may also suggest, but not require, that the patient explain or expand on something he has said. A good interviewer with a normally communicative patient should be able to gain much of the information he needs by attentive silence and facilitation. When the doctor senses that the patient is not speaking freely and clearly, however, he should consider making a confrontation.

Confrontation

In confrontation the interviewer describes to the patient something striking about his verbal or non-verbal behavior. Here the clinician exerts a little more control over the interview than he does in facilitation. Facilitation is a suggestion to the patient that he elaborate on a topic he has introduced. Confrontation directs the patient's attention to something that he may not be aware of—or, at best, be dimly aware of. As a result, a confrontation very often has the effect of introducing a new topic. Examples of confrontations are: "You look sad," "You seem frightened," "You sound angry," "I notice that you have been rubbing the back of your neck."

Like permitting a silence, confrontation poses a difficult problem for the beginning student of interviewing. Students are often self-conscious about using it. In ordinary casual social conversation one does not call the attention of the person with whom one is talking to striking aspects of his manner or behavior of which he is probably unaware. To do so would usually be considered impolite. Very often, too, confrontation is a hostile act; very often it is used in heated controversies. Since confrontation is not part of one's ordinary repertoire of social behaviors, one must develop through practice its use as an effective expression of sympathy or support during an interview.

One situation in which a confrontation is useful has been previously alluded to, that is, when the interviewer observes that the patient is having difficulty in providing information. Some of the possible reasons for this have already been discussed. It was suggested that if there is a pause during which the patient's discomfort has become evident and, perhaps, its nature revealed, a confrontation is in order unless the patient ends the silence by describing his difficulties. The form of the confrontation will depend on what the doctor has observed. Often useful are such comments as "You seem to be having a good deal of difficulty telling me about this" and "You appear quite uncomfortable." The patient who gives brief answers without elaborating may respond to "I notice you say very little except when I ask you questions." A common response is "Oh, I didn't know you wanted me to go on."

Note that the confrontations above describe how the patient appears to the interviewer. They are based on what he has *observed*. They do not make inferences about the patient's motives or his specific emotional state. It is of course possible that the interviewer has been incorrect in ascribing discomfort to the patient. In this case the remark will give the patient an opportunity to explain the difference between the clinician's perception of his behavior and his own. Such an explanation usually provides useful information.

The confrontation is not formulated as a question. At first glance, it might seem more efficient to ask, "Why are you uncomfortable?" or, "Why do you have so little to say?" There are several reasons for avoiding such questions. First, they assume that the physician is correct. A question puts more pressure on the patient to agree with the doctor than a mere statement of the doctor's observation does. Second, a direct question also requires that the patient make some reply. The patient may not have developed sufficient trust in the doctor to reveal the required information. He may make an evasive, partial, or even a false reply. Third, the patient may not know or be able to formulate the answer to the question. Feeling forced to reply, he gives a misleading or uninformative answer. The question "Why?" asks for a causal explanation. Many persons, especially among the lower socio-economic classes and the culturally deprived, do not think in terms of intra-psychic causes for their behavior or problems, and this is the realm of causation to which the doctor is usually referring. Even more important, a complete response to such a question would take the patient to his genetic endowment, his socialization from infancy to the present, the set of circumstances under which he is living, and what is happening in the interview situation. Asking why allows the patient to select some plausible "cause" out of that part of these data which are available to him. His explanation may very well be what he thinks the clinician believes or wishes to hear. This often leads to mutual acceptance of an explanation which appears plausible to the interviewer but which may or may not be either accurate or valid. In pointing out the patient's communicative difficulties the doctor is attempting less to discover their causes than to permit the patient to express the feelings he is then having. This expression may be sufficient in itself to permit the patient to continue; if not, the doctor may be able to assist the patient in continuing once he has listened to this expression.

Another situation in which confrontation is useful occurs when the patient's non-verbal behavior communicates something to the interviewer that the patient is not talking about. For example, a housewife may be describing some set of physical symptoms, and her doctor observes her dejected posture, sad look about her eyes, her low and monotonous voice, and her twisting fingers. By some remark like "It strikes me that you look very sad" the doctor responds to her non-verbal rather than her verbal communication. Slightly reddened eyes or trembling of the chin or lips may indicate that the patient is on the verge of tears. A sympathetic confrontation such as "You look as if you are about to cry" may offer the patient an opportunity to give vent to her feelings of despair by open weeping. This may have a most valuable therapeutic effect. Physicians in particular tend to avoid situations that encourage a patient to cry for fear the patient will later be ashamed or embarrassed about it. This fear very often stems from the doctor's own feelings about the shamefulness of crying. If the doctor responds to the weeping patient tactfully, it is very unlikely that the patient will feel ashamed or embarrassed.

It is appropriate, too, to confront a patient when his voice, posture, bodily movement, or facial expression betray emotions such as anger or anxiety. One can say, "I get the impression that you are angry," or, "You sound angry." To an anxious patient, one can say, "You look worried," or, "You seem tense," or one can remark on the behavior which betrays tension or anxiety by saying such things as "I notice you're chain-smoking" or "You're trembling." All such remarks tend to evoke a freer expression of feelings from the patient. Valuable information is derived and other needed information can be obtained more expeditiously after the patient's expression of his despair, fear, anger, or other strong feeling. Lastly, if the clinician handles the situation sensitively, the patient will feel increased trust and confidence.

A particularly appropriate time to confront a patient is when his verbal and non-verbal behavior are clearly incongruous. For example, a patient may speak about very sad things in an indifferent manner, about insults or gross injustice without displaying anger, or about comfortable circumstances and happy events in a mood of dejection. A comment on these discrepancies may lead to valuable information about the patient's difficulties and especially about his conflicts.

A confrontation is also appropriate when there are inconsistencies in the patient's story. This almost always leads to valuable information.

There are a few cautions to be stated about confrontations. In ordinary conversation, when we speak of confronting someone, we often mean a hostile accusation. This term often has an unpleasant and unnecessary connotation of anger, even though there are many types of helpful and positive confrontations. When confrontations are made in an interview they should reflect sympathetic interest in the patient. Sometimes the interviewer's irritation with some behavior of the patient may be the cue that calls this behavior to his attention, but it is his interest in this peculiarity of behavior and in furthering the goals of the interview that should prompt and be expressed in the confrontation. A second caution concerns the overuse of confrontation. Even though the patient is confronted in a sympathetic manner, he may feel criticized if he is confronted too often. Confrontations can develop a nagging quality. No more than one or two confrontations about the same or related observations are appropriate in any interview.

Questions

The question, which could be called directive evocation,[6] requests information and specifies the area of information desired in the response. This is the highest use of authority and it exercises the greatest degree of control thus far discussed. Open-ended questions vary in the degree of authority they represent depending on how closely they specify the area in which the reply is expected.

Questions that require a very specific answer are rarely appropriate if the interviewer does not know how he will use the information in arriving at a decision. If direct questions are properly phrased, answers will most often be brief but high in information content.

Even greater control is exerted when the question is so phrased that a yes or no answer is called for. A similar form is the multiple choice query in which the interviewer specifies a list of specific replies he expects the patient to choose from: "Does this pain come on before, after, or during meals?" These two types of questions we may term *check-list questions* since they verbally offer the kind of question which may be answered by checking off a pre-printed response on a questionnaire.

Check list questions are generally to be avoided in an interview. Both types tend to stop the interchange. The patient "checks-off" the reply and waits for the next question. Furthermore, both types tend to suggest that the interviewer is not interested in information which does not fall into the categories provided and expects the patient to "pigeon hole" his reply categorically. More communicative patients may overcome this suggestion and provide relevant information not requested, but the interviewer should not rely on this when formulating questions. It is particularly difficult to create good multiple choice questions spontaneously. The categories should be exhaustive and mutually exclusive. If all possible alternatives are not offered, bias is introduced. If all alternatives are presented the question is likely to be so complex that it confuses the patient. Multiple choice questions are, therefore, best given in written form. Questions represent the interviewing behavior most likely to produce biased information. A discussion of ways to avoid bias will be found in Chapter 4.

At what points in the interview is it wise to use direct questions? The first is any time one cannot get needed information with a lower degree of authority. The second is when the broad outlines of the story have emerged and specific information about details is needed. These include the review of systems, inquiry into past illnesses, and parts of the mental status examination. Chapter 4 will deal with these aspects of the interview.

Direction, the highest use of control, refers to statements or actions that indicate, instruct, or demand of the other what he should do in such a way that an expected compliance is clearly indicated. Directions to speak, such as "Tell me more about that," exert the full force of the doctor's authority. However, the direction cited does not limit the range of information that the patient will give to anything like the degree that a direct and highly specific question will do so. Thus, directions, too, can allow a patient considerable latitude in what he says, though little latitude in the topic he speaks about.

Somewhat less control than with either questions or directions is exercised when the interviewer makes a *suggestion*. A suggestion is a subtle direction or advice which may guide the patient's thinking or behavior. Because of the authority of the clinician it will have much more effect on the patient than the same words would have in a different setting. Suggestion is the commonest way of biasing information, for this reason. This can be done in several ways. One is by the wording of the question. Another is by shifting topics, which may say to the patient, "That's not important—no more about that." It can also be done by interpreting what the patient has said, or by mentioning a tentative diagnosis. Suggesting a pattern of pain or a symptom must be avoided in diagnostic interviewing. However, suggestion may be helpful in treatment; it is probably the basis of the placebo effect.

Support and Reassurance

In the first part of this chapter, we mentioned that trust and confidence in the clinician is built when, among other things, the patient is offered support. This is also true of reassurance, when appropriate and correctly timed. The clinician's ability to be appropriately supportive and reassuring helps create an atmosphere in which the patient is encouraged to communicate. It also helps to promote the continuity of the relationship.

Support refers to any act which communicates the interviewer's interest in, liking for, or understanding of the patient or which promotes a feeling of security in the relationship. Examples of supportive statements are: "I understand" and "That must have been very upsetting." A summary of what the patient has just said that conveys a sympathetic comprehension is supportive.

One of the most important times to express support is after the patient has expressed strong feeling. After a confrontation to which the patient has responded with weeping, or the expression of hitherto tightly controlled fear or anger, support is most important. It increases the solidarity of the relationship and helps the patient to continue his account.

It must be clearly understood that supportive words without a supportive attitude on the part of the interviewer will sound hollow and will fail to accomplish their intended purpose. Without a genuine interest in the patient, a feeling of friendliness, and a desire to be helpful, supportive words are simply not supportive.

Reassurance includes words or acts which tend in the direction of restoring the patient's sense of well-being, worthiness, or confidence. When patients are very frightened, a reassuring remark may have a remarkably helpful effect. As with support, if the words are of reassurance but the clinician's attitude does not convey reassurance, the attempt will fail. To be effective, reassurance must be based on evidence or fact and be genuine. Clichés are rarely reassuring.

Since reassurance depends on acceptance of the doctor's authority, reassurance should not be given in a way that creates unreasonable expectations. Staying close to fact is the best way of avoiding this. The clinician can reassure by citing what he has learned up to that point and how it can be interpreted. On the other hand, to state, "Everything will be all right," or, "There is nothing to fear," unless the evidence clearly supports such a statement is a poor use of reassurance. "You are making satisfactory progress" is reassuring only if it is based on good evidence that the patient can understand.

The open-ended interview, in summary, represents a style of interviewing that adds features of the interviewing approaches characteristic of psychiatric and social casework interviewing to the traditional medical interview. The medical interview emphasizes data collection and aims for high efficiency in gathering detailed data within limited time periods. The aspects added from mental health interviewing include greater attention to rapport and to the development of the clinician-patient relationship and an attempt to facilitate the *emergence* of facts rather than their *extraction* from the patient, thereby creating the opportunity for less biased and more relevant information, verbal and non-verbal. It relies on a differential use of the clinician's authority, never using more authority than is required to get the needed data, and on the ability of the interviewer, through appropriate support and reassurance, to express his interest in helping the patient.

REFERENCES

1. Hollender, M. H., *The Psychology of Medical Practice*. Philadelphia: W. B. Saunders, 1958.
2. Gill, M., R. Newman, and F. C. Redlich, *The Initial Interview in Psychiatric Practice*. New York: International Universities Press, 1954.
3. Enelow, A. J., L. M. Adler, and P. Manning, "A Supervised Psychotherapy Course for Practicing Physicians," *Journal of Medical Education*, 39, 140-46, 1964.
4. Adler, L. M., and A. J. Enelow, "A Scale To Measure Psychotherapy Interactions." Paper read at the annual meeting of the American Psychiatric Association, May 8, 1964, Los Angeles, California.
5. Adler, L. M., and A. J. Enelow, "An Instrument To Measure Skill in Diagnostic Interviewing: A Teaching and Evaluation Tool," *Journal of Medical Education*, 41:281-288, 1966.
6. Enelow, A. J., and M. Wexler, *Psychiatry in the Practice of Medicine*. New York: Oxford University Press, 1966.
7. Payne, S. L., *The Art of Asking Questions*. Princeton, N.J.: Princeton University Press, 1951.

4

OBTAINING ADDITIONAL SPECIFIC INFORMATION

Direct Questioning, System Review, and Physical Examination

At several points in every medical interview, the physician must intervene to obtain specific information about a problem that has been tentatively identified. This may require asking direct questions. As we previously commented, interviewers frequently resort to direct questions too early in the course of the clinical interview. Physicians in particular tend to have difficulty refraining from prematurely testing a possible diagnosis suggested by a problem cue. By intervening too early in the course of the interview with questions, the physician easily destroys the patient's initiative in telling his story. A great deal of specific information can be obtained from the patient's spontaneous account, making it possible to ask fewer highly directive questions with their resultant constriction of range of information. Direct questions can then be used to fill in the gaps.

1 QUESTIONING DURING THE OPEN-ENDED PHASE OF THE INTERVIEW

While direct questioning of the patient should usually occur only after the patient seems to have completed telling his own story spontaneously, direct questioning may be indicated much earlier with the patient who rambles and repeats or strays away repeatedly into unrelated or unimportant topics. Questions which seek clarification of topics the patient has just volunteered, such as the precise time sequence of events, the exact location of a described phenomenon, the exact amount of a drug taken, and similar questions, will usually be well tolerated during a patient's spontaneous account if they do not interrupt him and are introduced at an appropriate pause. Such questions may heighten his responsiveness and increase his efforts to be precise if they can be seen as evidence of the physician's interest in gathering all relevant data.

A word of caution is in order here. Questioning for clarification and to add significant details can shut off communication if it is directed to a topic about which the patient is defensive or has a great deal of conflict. If the interviewer feels that a given topic may be such a conflict-laden area, it is best to save that detailed inquiry for a later time in the interview. This is wise for several reasons. For one, it permits the patient to develop some feeling of trust in the interviewer, if he is able to. For another it avoids a possible premature cessation of all communication, as occurred in the following example.

> A student was interviewing a patient who had been admitted to the hospital because of severe chest pain that was thought to be a possible myocardial infarction. The patient had a long history of frequent attacks of angina pectoris. During the spontaneous account of his difficulties, the patient said he had been taking 5 or 6 nitroglycerine tablets daily and frequently took Demerol tablets. At an appropriate pause, the student began an inquiry into the frequency with which he took Demerol, the dose, and so forth. At first the patient supplied the information, then, visibly stiffening, ceased to do so. He asked the student to terminate the interview, stating, "You're asking me too many questions."

2 AVOIDING BIAS IN DIRECT INQUIRY

Regardless of the time or reason for introducing direct questions, good interviewing technique requires that direct inquiry be conducted in a manner which does not bias the resulting communication. The principle is this: accuracy in communication is facilitated when the interviewer does not suggest responses he expects or approves by the wording of his questions or by his demeanor, tone of voice or other non-verbal communication. The interviewer's manner can be a source of bias. Facial expressions or gestures which express moral approval or disapproval, surprise, or greatly accentuated interest or attention will influence what the patient tells or does not tell. The wording of the interviewer's communication can also reveal his own biases and thereby influence the patient's account.

Designers of public opinion surveys have made a careful study of ways of avoiding bias in wording questions.[1] One of these is to avoid emotionally loaded words. For example, "Is she a good baby?" is less likely to elicit accurate information than "How often does the baby cry?" "Have you ever had a pregnancy terminated?" is preferable to "Have you ever had an abortion?"

In general, the more open-ended the question the more likely the answer will be accurate. In other words, one should avoid suggesting an expected answer and permit the patient to formulate his own reply. Ask "When does the pain come on?" rather than "Does the pain come on right after meals?"

As the interviewer seeks more detailed information, it becomes increasingly difficult to formulate open-ended questions. Therefore as questions become highly specific, alternatives should be stated. From behavioral science research on question wording, it has been learned that a question like "Does the pain come on right after meals?" will elicit more "yes" responses than will a question worded like "Does the pain come on right after meals, or do you notice it at other times?" In so wording a question, one should give each alternative equal weight, as in "Does exertion bring on the pain, or do you notice it at times when you have not been exerting yourself?" Even adding "or not?" to a single alternative will reduce the likelihood of a biased response to some degree.

It is most important to formulate questions in a way that does not suggest an expected answer or pattern of pain. Thus, "Does the pain stay in one place or does it move or travel?" is a good question. "Does the pain shoot down your leg?" is more likely to bias the patient's account. Confrontation may be used to avoid the introduction of bias. For example, if a patient repeatedly rubs some part of his body such as his knee, it is better to use confrontation: "I notice that you're rubbing your knee," than to ask, "Does your knee hurt?"

Another point at which there is danger of introducing bias is when facilitating the patient's communication by summarizing what he has just said. Here one may unthinkingly introduce an inference about what he has said, or reflect a personal judgment about it, either critical or approving.

The timing of questions and of shifts in topic can introduce bias also. It is important, therefore, to avoid interpretations or suggestions about the nature of the problem during information-gathering phases of the interview. Also, one should not pursue a specific line of inquiry longer than really necessary or to the exclusion of other unexplored areas. Excessive and highly detailed concentration on one area or line of inquiry will often convince the patient that there *must* be something there; otherwise the clinician would not be so intensely preoccupied with that area. In the same vein, rapid shifts in a line of inquiry may suggest to the patient that a given theme is not significant before it has been explored. Similarly, shifting from topic to topic and repeatedly returning to them can be confusing to the patient and reduce his accuracy of reporting. In brief, stay with a given line of inquiry as long as necessary to get all needed information, but no longer. Questions should always be framed for the specific patient being interviewed, taking into account his language skills, social and cultural background, and style of communication. With all patients, one should use simple, concise non-technical language.

3 DEVELOPING A LINE OF INQUIRY

When the clinician decides to seek specific information, it is best obtained by gradually restricting the open-endedness of a series of questions presented to the patient. This is done by beginning with a most general and exploratory question pertinent to the body area or the topic in which the specific answer is sought. For example, in reviewing the respiratory system, if one wishes to find out whether the patient has pain in the upper right anterior area of the chest and whether it is made worse by respiration, an appropriate sequence of questions might be:

1. "How are your chest and lungs?"
2. (If symptoms are mentioned) "Could you please describe the discomfort (or pain)?"
3. "Where is the pain?" or "Could you please show me where the pain is?"
4. "Is the pain always the same or does it change?"
5. (If it changes) "What kind of things affect the pain?"
6. (If deep breathing is not mentioned) "Does deep breathing affect it at all?"

At any point in this sequence of questions, the patient might respond with all of the information, in his own words, that the physician is seeking. In fact, he might add a whole set of new and important associated data. If he has responded to the first question with all the needed information, the skilled interviewer asks no more, to avoid the implication that he is interested primarily in pain or the effects of breathing. This encourages the patient to respond to other relatively open-ended questions with data that tends to be uninfluenced and unprejudiced by the clinician's inquiry.

If the patient responds in the negative to a relatively broad question, such as the first one listed above, the topic can be dropped at this point and the interviewer can move on to another area or topic of possible interest, particularly if the patient has demonstrated an easy responsiveness and the ability to communicate information effectively. If, however, the specific bit of information being sought, positive or negative, is of major importance in testing a given diagnostic possibility, it may be wise to pursue the line of questioning despite a negative response to the first one. One might go on to ask, "Do you have pain anywhere in the chest?" and even though this evokes a negative reply, ask "Do you ever have discomfort in breathing?" While the wording of these questions encourages positive replies, this is the conservative approach in this circumstance. Finally, if the patient has denied symptoms and this is of crucial importance in establishing the diagnosis, it is justifiable to conclude with: "Then you are having no discomfort in your chest or lungs. Is that correct or have I misunderstood?" The exercise of clinical judgment is required in making the decision about how far to pursue specific information. It is based upon knowledge of the potential importance of the specific information being sought, as well as evaluation of the patient and his responses in the interview up to that point. Obviously, with a suggestible patient, it is best not to pursue information to the extent described. With sensitivity of the issues involved, this judgment is acquired with experience.

4 DIRECT QUESTIONING AFTER THE OPEN-ENDED PHASE OF THE INTERVIEW

Each symptom or bodily discomfort, whether reported by the patient spontaneously or elicited by the interviewer, requires specific qualifying information in order to be evaluated. It is usually best to delay inquiry into this qualifying information until after the patient's spontaneous account. Any necessary information that is not supplied by the patient should also be sought later, during the stage of the interview in which direct questions are being asked in order to fill in gaps. The qualifying information needed includes the following.

1. Location. Where is it experienced? If pain, does it radiate? If so, where? Under what circumstances does it do so?
2. Quality. What does it feel like? Is it dull or sharp, cutting, aching, throbbing, grinding? Other adjectives that may be used are "pressure," "crushing," "like a vise or band." If the discomfort is a limitation of function, as difficulty in breathing, a similar description of the character of the experience is needed.
3. Intensity. The terms the patient will use represent a mixture of

subjective response to the pain as well as degree of severity. Though the description will range from mild to very severe or even unbearable, it should be evaluated in terms of the patient's personality or temperament. One man's severe pain is another's mild pain.

4. Quantitative aspects. How many? How often? How much? How big? Each of these may be applicable, depending on the type of discomfort or symptom reported.
5. Time of onset, duration, and frequency. If several symptoms are reported, what is their chronological relationship to each other, if any?
6. Setting. Under what circumstances does the symptom occur? Can it be related to the patient's location, his physical environment, or his social environment?
7. Aggravation and alleviation. Does anything make it worse or better?
8. Are there clearly related symptoms, limitations of function, or subjective responses, such as sensations of heat or cold, anxiety, depression, dizziness, faintness?
9. Has the patient taken medication or made other attempts to modify the symptoms chemically or physically?

Having reconstructed the patient's clinical problems and current symptoms beginning with their onset and having identified the course of the present illness, the interviewer should turn to the past medical history. Once again, the preferred approach is to begin with an open-ended inquiry. "How has your health been before this difficulty began?" is a good opening question. The usual response is a general one which requires elaboration. If the patient says something like, "Pretty good," or "Fair," the interviewer should be facilitative. "Pretty good?" as a response will usually elicit qualifying data. If necessary, one can increase the specificity of questions until periods of ill health, as well as adequacy of general functioning during periods of good health, have been described. Ongoing problems, such as allergies, may call for a specific inquiry. For previous illnesses, the patient's report of a given diagnosis should not be accepted at face value. It is better to try to identify it from the account of onset, course, duration, type of treatment, and residual symptoms or functional limitation following the illness. This part of the interview will usually make it possible to place the present illness in the context of general health and previous adult illnesses and injuries.

The patient will usually not, however, give specific information about childhood health. If he does not, the interviewer begins again: "How was your health as a child?" Following the procedure of gradual increase in specificity of questions, one can inquire about specific illnesses, and finally, if need be, inquire about important childhood illnesses by name, as well as specific ones that might have a bearing on the present problem.

Other areas to be filled in with specific inquiries include the health status of the other family members and the relationships of the family members to each other and to the family as a unit.

If the patient's social history and the details of his current life situation with regard to family work, life style, current emotional problems, and reactions to present stresses upon him have not emerged by this time, specific inquiries should now be directed to this. A well-conducted interview will usually be characterized by the patient giving this information in context as he describes his present illness and past health.

5 DIRECT QUESTIONING TO DEVELOP NEW AREAS OF INFORMATION

Direct questioning of patients is of two types. The first is that related to one or more of the problems the patient has already presented during the more open-ended phase of the interview, and the second is that designed to uncover other data or problems the patient has not remembered or has not described previously. Direct questioning about known problems should be carried out first and in order of the apparent relative importance of the problems. These questions should be designed to provide the clinician with a complete picture of these problems, in the light of his knowledge of the probable or possible disease processes involved. As always, the principle of asking the broadest questions first, followed by increasingly directed and specific questions, should be observed. This is a skill that can be attained only with practice. This requires a self-consciousness about one's phrasing of questions as a beginner. With experience, it becomes automatic.

Questions designed to elicit information the patient has not given voluntarily are commonly called the *Review of Systems* in the conventional medical record. This is usually taught as a list of fifty to a hundred questions covering cardinal disease manifestations of the body systems. In the name of thoroughness they are usually asked in check-list fashion of all patients as part of the so-called "complete work-up." No work-up can be truly complete, and much time is wasted by medical students and house officers in pursuit of this mythical ideal. It is our belief that if one tried instead for a better grasp of basic interviewing skills, the quality of the information available in medical records would be noticeably improved. Medical information can be obtained in check-list fashion more economically by a non-physician interviewer or health aide, by the use of a self-administered questionnaire, or by a computer assisted data-gathering system. While useful to the physician, such data may be especially valuable for other medical purposes, such as health screening. It should not be a primary component of a physician's interview. Physicians should take advantage of their ability to do what cannot be done by fixed question lists: to listen to and interpret in the light of one's knowledge of disease and of the patient, the uninfluenced story of a patient's problems as he sees them.

Nevertheless, it is useful to give the patient an opportunity to recall and describe complaints and observations not volunteered previously in the interview. The basic technique involved is the same as that already described for questioning the patient for amplification of information already obtained. A general, open-ended question, directed only enough to indicate the organ, system, area of the body, or function to which you wish the patient to attend, is asked first. If the patient replies negatively or gives only inconsequential information, the interviewer may move on. The next similar question is then posed. In certain areas, and with certain patients, second and third more specific questions may be asked. For example, in questioning a patient about possible cardiac dysfunction or disease, the first question might be: "Have you ever had any problems with your heart, or not?" If the reply is "no" it might be appropriate to ask a fifty-year-old obese male: "Do you have any shortness of breath when you are exerting yourself?" and "Do you have any pain in your chest brought on by hard work or exercise?" Additional specific questions may be asked based upon the level of suspicion created by other aspects of the situation. These would include the circumstances in which the patient is seen, his appearance, and what he has said earlier in the interview. A rote list of perfunctory questions should be avoided at all costs. On the other hand, each clinician tends to develop his own system-directed inquiries which he can use when needed.

What is usually termed the system review is best thought of as an organizing device and an aid to the memory. That is, after obtaining an account of the present illness and the past health history as an adult and child and after filling in significant gaps through direct inquiry it is well to consider whether all organ systems and areas of the body that could be of relevance to the assessment of the present state of health or illness have been covered. Inquiries can then be made, if indicated, either during the physical examination or just prior to undertaking it. The same systematic order of conducting the physical examination supplies the major headings for this phase of data collection. A well-conducted interview will usually have brought out most of the information. The remainder is easily obtained just prior to examining each system or area.

6 THE MENTAL STATUS EXAMINATION

It is only of academic interest to debate whether the mental status examination is part of the so-called Review of Systems or part of the physical examination. But no clinical examination of a patient is complete without one. It is also a moot point as to whether to assign it to the interview or to the physical examination. In fact, it cannot be assigned to either because it belongs to both. Assessment of mental status goes on throughout the period of time that the clinician and the patient are together. In the case of some patients, particularly children and those who are guarded, it may be necessary to interview other family members in order to complete the examination. In many, if not most, instances very few specific inquiries need be made since it can be easily ascertained whether or not the areas of mental functioning with which the examiner is concerned are within normal limits. This means, however, that the examiner has had these areas of mental functioning in mind throughout the interview. While the patient tells his story, the interviewer concerns himself with both content and process. He listens to what the patient says and how he says it. If he then gets evidence that the mental status needs closer scrutiny, he can make the necessary inquiries.

The areas to be examined in a thorough mental status examination are: appearance and behavior, speech, mood, thought content, perception, and orientation.

Appearance and Behavior

As the patient enters the room, the examiner notes his posture or carriage, dress, facial expression, and attitude. The depressed patient, for example, usually looks sad or washed-out, moves slowly, and appears to be tentative or unsure. When seated, his shoulders will droop and his facial expression will be characterized by a downturned mouth and a bleak or unhappy look. On the other hand, the anxious patient will transmit a look of apprehension, often will be restless or even tremulous and may perspire freely. One should note the patient's dress, the feeling tone transmitted by his facial expression (anger, bewilderment, fear, blandness, sadness, and so forth), his attitude toward the interviewer, and the interviewer's response.

Speech

How the patient talks will give important diagnostic clues. Tone of voice, inflection, volume (if very loud or very soft), continuity (does the patient speak rapidly, slowly, haltingly? Are there long periods of silence?), and organization (coherence, logicality, ability to give an account without rambling into unrelated irrelevancies or excessive detail) are the important features to note.

Mood

How does the patient feel? If he does not tell you spontaneously, an inquiry is in order. A confrontation about observed evidence of a disturbance in mood is the preferred approach when possible. Some patients are aware of feeling depressed, or anxious, or of having disturbing fluctuations of mood and freely volunteer this information. Others will not speak about it until they are asked or confronted with your observations about their mood. And there are patients who have disturbances of mood but deny this, as though it might just "go away" if they pretend it's not there. For this reason the interviewer should check his own impression of the patient's mood against the patient's description. Hints about suicidal tendencies should be followed up and thoroughly explored. Other disturbances of mood that may be reported are feelings of unreality or of detachment. And some patients will state, "I don't feel anything," a very distressing state akin to severe and chronic depression.

Thought Content

What are the patient's pre-occupations, and how realistic do they appear to be? Does he have obsessions (repetitive, often unpleasant but uncontrollable thoughts), compulsions (feeling compelled to perform repetitive acts), delusions, hallucinations?

Perception and Orientation

In the usual diagnostic interview with a general medical patient this is not a detailed examination. If, however, it becomes apparent that the patient has serious psychiatric problems, the examination of the patient's cognitive function should be carried out in detail. Cognitive testing consists of asking a series of formal questions borrowed from diagnostic psychological tests. These are described in standard textbooks of psychiatry. In the non-psychiatric patient, it is necessary to note only whether the patient is oriented (that is, aware of who he is, where he is, the date, and time), has the ability to pay attention to what is happening, and is capable of ordinary concentration. One should also note defects of memory, ability to do abstract reasoning, evidence of reasonably good or of poor judgment, and adequacy of perception—visual, auditory, and tactile.

While it is very likely that defects of perception and orientation will become apparent in the course of a well-conducted interview, one can be misled by patients who have brain damage and who confabulate. Such patients will fill in the gaps in their defective memory with facts and details manufactured on the spot. If these are not blatantly self-contradictory, the examiner may not recognize them as confabulations. If the interviewer has any clue that brain damage, such as from chronic alcoholism, is part of the problem, it is well to inquire directly about the date, time, and place. Such a patient commonly will not be able to state the day, month, and year; nor will he be able to account satisfactorily for recent periods of time.

7 INTERVIEWING DURING THE PHYSICAL EXAMINATION

Communication with the patient should not be allowed to lapse during performance of the physical examination. Silence on the part of the physician as he examines may be regarded as ominous by the apprehensive patient. If the patient feels that silence is expected by the physician, he may not respond if, as a result of some maneuver of the physical examination, he recalls a fact he would like to add to the information already given. The physical examination should be orderly and comprehensive, requirements best satisfied by employing an unvarying basic routine. The inexperienced physician may find it difficult to divide his attention between what he is doing and observing and what the patient is saying that might be of importance. However, the examiner should learn to continue speaking with the patient while examining him if for no other reason than to relieve tension and maintain open lines of communication with the patient. This is still another reason for using the time of the physical examination to complete the organ- and system-directed inquiry, previously described as the Review of Systems. It is most appropriate to do it at this time because the inquiry and the physical examination, properly performed, mutually reinforce each other. The questions with the related examination procedure strongly stimulate recall by the patient. The patient's responses help to direct the physician's examining procedure and his interpretations of what he observes. Time is also saved. If the physician does question the patient as he examines, he should of course use the technique we have emphasized of asking first the most open-ended question pertinent to the area under investigation, followed by increasingly specific questions as necessary. Timing of the questions is crucial; the first question should always be posed *before* beginning to examine a given area. The patient will then respond while the area is being examined, unless silence is needed to permit auscultation. In that case, permit the patient to answer before asking him for the period of silence needed while you listen. If the first question about a given organ or system is asked during or after examining it, the patient may take this to mean that a significant abnormality has been encountered. This creates anxiety and the patient is then likely to be more interested in finding out what you have discovered than in providing information. While it is difficult to learn to maintain the proper timing relationship of questioning and examining, with questions just leading the related examination procedure, it is a most useful skill that can be acquired by experience if it is regularly practiced.

8 EXAMINING THE ANXIOUS PATIENT

If a patient is becoming visibly anxious during the physical examination, in spite of the precautions noted, it is appropriate to give reassurance periodically with casual comments on the normality of certain of the findings. If a patient's level of anxiety is rising, it almost always inhibits his communication. If you find that open-ended questions yield progressively less information from the patient and more and more highly specific questions are required, it is reasonable to assume that the patient is becoming increasingly anxious. It is well to interrupt the examination at this point and inquire into this. The line of questioning may have been too highly directive. The patient may be becoming anxious or depressed. Something may have suggested to the patient that you are not really interested in him or are not to be trusted. Or, you may have unwittingly provoked anxiety by a variety of unintentional errors of omission or commission. For example, when a patient is alone and unclothed in an austere examining room and has a prolonged wait for the doctor, he will very likely become anxious and depressed or angry. It is always important to examine such a situation critically. The preferred approach is to confront the patient supportively with your observations about his communication and manner. Very often, then, he will tell you what is creating the inhibition. Often, too, some information or reassurance can be given that will put the patient much more at ease. Interviewing the anxious patient is discussed in Chapter 6.

This chapter, together with Chapter 3, comprises a description of how to obtain valid, precise, and reliable data with high information content from patients. It is written from the point of view of the clinician. The reader's understanding of the interviewing process will be enhanced by a study of Chapter 10, "The Social Context of the Clinical Interview."

REFERENCE

1. Payne, S. L., *The Art of Asking Questions*. Princeton, N.J.: Princeton University Press, 1951.

5

THE PROBLEM-ORIENTED MEDICAL RECORD

1 INTRODUCTION

Medical students and house officers commonly regard medical record keeping as drudgery of high order. Practicing physicians, after several years of experience, usually discover the value of their own records, at least in terms of time saved and improved efficiency. Some even find in their records a source of self-evaluation and the basis for a higher quality of professional practice. Nevertheless, current medical record keeping is not at a generally high level.

Most physicians, beginning and experienced, regard the medical record as primarily an archival document, a historical record to be consulted from time to time when memory fails. This chapter will present a concept of the medical record which is quite different: the medical record as an integral part of the clinical problem-solving process. In this role, the record becomes a dynamic device which closely reflects the patient's status and is important in the delivery of optimal patient care. Of course, problem-oriented records still serve the function of documentation. In fact they are enriched in this respect because they exhibit the *processes* of patient care as well as the "facts of the case." The value of such records in auditing the quality of medical care, a practice which we feel will become universal in the United States in the near future, is obvious. But for the present a discussion of the format of the traditional medical record is necessary, and it may provide a useful perspective. This conventional record form will still be required of students and house officers in many institutions for some time; changes in long-standing practices take place slowly. (Sample form on pages 86-91.)

The Conventional Medical Record

The classical medical record contains the patient's history in six parts, physical findings described by organ systems, initial laboratory data, and a variable pattern for the formulation of diagnoses, diagnostic planning, and therapeutic proposals. These elements are recorded in the initial evaluation of a patient in the sequence indicated by the numbers in Table I, below.

The historical record is primarily in chronological sequence, with the data about one or more illnesses flowing together. The information recorded is categorized rather rigidly and arbitrarily; current findings and historical facts are usually sharply separated.

TABLE I

Historical Data	*Current Data*	*Problem Statements*	*Proposed Solutions*
1. Chief Complaint	7. Physical Findings	9. Formulation	11. Diagnostic Plans
2. Present Illness	8. Initial Laboratory Data	10. Diagnoses	12. Therapeutic Plans
3. Past Medical History			
4. Social Psychological History			
5. Family History			
6. Review of Systems			

Follow-up notes in the classical record vary widely in style, content and relevance to current medical practice. In general, they record additional facts and observations as they accrue. The notes usually deal with all concurrent disease processes. Sometimes these notes accumulate in different and unrelated sections of the clinical record as reports of various special services or laboratories. Unfortunately progress notes do not commonly record an emerging synthesis and resolution of the patient's problems. Following the threads of multiple, long-term, and complex illnesses through such a record is usually a major undertaking.

The origins of this record format remain obscure. The format was apparently well established in its current form on the Harvard services of the Boston City Hospital in the early 1920's under Dr. Francis Peabody, who strongly emphasized the importance of social, psychological, and family historical data in the medical record.* The format has acquired something of a stylized literary quality in many medical centers, and many generations of medical students have been judged by their mastery of it. In particular, the list of questions that appears under the heading of Review of Systems is asked of all patients, regardless of their pertinence, and has become highly institutionalized.

Defects in the Conventional Medical Record

The conventional medical record format has a number of obvious, if recently recognized, defects. Beginning the document with a single chief complaint subtly suggests the outmoded concept that a single diagnosis will "explain" the patient's illness. It forces patient and physician to assign primacy to one of several possible concurrent illnesses. It is frequently difficult to determine at what point in time to begin the narrative description of the present illness or illnesses if the present episode is clearly or even remotely

* The authors are indebted to Dr. G. O. Broun, Sr., Department of Medicine, St. Louis University School of Medicine, for an opportunity to examine medical records created in this era and for his comments on Dr. Peabody's influence on the content of the medical record.

related to an incident in the past. More seriously, the classical record commonly does not disentangle those elements of multiple, etiologically unrelated but interacting illnesses that occur simultaneously, even though it is clear that the skilled physician does just this as his first step in processing the data he receives directly from the patient.

There is little reason to segregate information under social, psychological, or family headings when it is of direct pertinence to one or more of the patient's past or present illnesses. The many questions of the usual Review of Systems serve more as an *aide de memoire* for the physician; particularly when the patient responds in the negative, they hardly need to be recorded as evidence of his assiduousness.

The most serious criticism of the classical medical record lies in the rather arbitrary separation of historical aspects from the related current physical and laboratory findings of a disease process, which taken together, form the very basis of clinical diagnosis. Current records frequently leave the reader puzzled about how the formulations and diagnoses were reached. Should not all of the kinds of data pertinent to an identifiable problem be considered together, along with its formulation and related diagnostic and therapeutic projections? The problem-oriented medical record (P.O.R.), introduced by Lawrence Weed, has this as its primary goal.[1, 2, 3] This basic concept can be extended into other aspects of patient care to great advantage.[4]

2 PRINCIPLES OF THE PROBLEM-ORIENTED RECORD

The Problem List

The first requirement of the problem-oriented record is development of a well-defined list of problems which encompasses all the significant difficulties the patient is experiencing. This list of problems will include those which are presented as "complaints" by the patient, as well as those detected by the physician in the course of physical and laboratory examinations. Creation of an inclusive problem list requires that a useful *Data Base* be available first, since analysis of these data is required before the actual record is created. This is in contrast to the commonly held idea that the data should not be analyzed until they have been recorded in narrative and descriptive form.

Problem Titles and the Master Problem List

The master problem list is the first element of the P.O.R. The problem list must be comprehensive; that is, eventually all of the pertinent data available should be assignable to one or more of the problems that have been identified. Relatively short, informative titles should be assigned to the problems and they should be serially numbered. The same titles and numbers should be used in the future by all observers who write in that particular record.

An effective knowledge of differential diagnosis is essential in preparing the problem list. A problem sufficiently well analyzed and supported by data to permit a specific diagnosis can be identified by that diagnosis. However, it is not necessary to have reached an unequivocal diagnosis in order to identify and label a problem. If a diagnosis is not yet evident, the problem may be identified by the primary symptom or by a physical or laboratory finding. Then, as further data accumulate and a better analysis becomes possible, the title or description of the problem can be changed when a diagnosis is reached. The number of the problem should not be changed, even if it is a short-term acute and non-recurring problem that has been resolved.

The capacity to identify as a problem a related group of data which cannot yet be analyzed in terms of a specific diagnosis is one of the major strengths of the problem-oriented record. This should eliminate the confusing practice of listing a very large number of differential diagnostic possibilities in the formulation, each preceded by a question mark, when a problem is identifiable but not yet diagnosable.

Assigning Data to the Identified Problems

The process of identifying the patient's problems and assigning the available data to them is the most difficult and intellectually demanding task involved in diagnosis, particularly when two or more independent but interacting disease processes are involved. Indeed, it remains one of the principal unsolved problems of generalized computer-based diagnosis. The computer is unable to carry out this process because the rules which govern it cannot be described precisely and comprehensively. Once accurate assignment of medical diagnostic data to a list of problems has been accomplished by a physician, however, computer-assisted diagnosis becomes much more feasible. Another reason for students and physicians to learn to organize data in the P.O.R. format is that it will facilitate future medical record storage and retrieval methods employing large-scale computers or other automated data-processing techniques.

When the problem list is first developed, it is generally wiser to formulate too many problems rather than too few. Problems listed separately, with the beginning assumption that they are independent, will tend to converge into a single problem statement as additional data become available if in fact they are related. Experience seems to show that disentanglement of several problems falsely considered to be a single problem is somewhat more difficult to achieve. Yet obviously, assuming an excessive number of problems initially defeats much of the record's usefulness in problem-solving. The ideal problem list covers all of the patient's significant illnesses and difficulties, with each of the identified problems etiologically independent of the others.

Revising the Problem List

When a new problem is added to the list as the evaluation of the patient proceeds, it should be assigned a new problem title and number. If the new problem replaces one or more problems of the previous list, these should be closed on the list with some such notation as "replaced by problem #____." Division of what was thought to be a single problem into two (or more) problems is again best accomplished by the assignment of two new descriptions and numbers with these notations on the problem list: Old problem title—"replaced by problems #___ & #___." New problem titles—"formerly part of problem #___." Another similar technique of managing the problem list with somewhat different conventions is given in the outline found at the end of this chapter.

When a problem is resolved by appropriate treatment or other intervention, the problem list is revised by adding an entry about the nature of the outcome, such as "recovered." If a patient dies, the principal cause of death should be so identified on the master problem list.

The date when a problem is first formulated should also be noted on the master problem list. Thus, as new problems are recognized, they will appear in chronological order on the problem list with serial numbers. A problem that was closed in the past when the patient was thought to have recovered but later recurs should be added again to the master list with the previous title and number and with a new date and the notation "recurrent."

Data Not Assignable to a Problem

In the course of a medical interview and examination of a patient, certain data are obtained that are pertinent to but do not constitute a part of a "problem" in the strict sense. The test of such data is whether or not they can possibly be regarded as a problem which may require a solution to help the patient. For example, statements about the patient's race, age, sex, marital status, current and past family structure, height and weight if in the normal range, age, hair and eye color, habits, occupations past and present, and a wide variety of other life experiences are a legitimate part of the data base but do not identify specific problems. Many of these items *may* be pertinent, directly or indirectly, to a problem that has been identified on the basis of other data. For example, the fact that the patient is a male is important if the diagnosis of hemophilia is being considered under a problem title such as Bleeding Tendency.

These data may also be pertinent to problems encountered in the patient's future care.

Patient Profile

It is also important to record a characterization of the patient, largely in behavioral terms, and to describe in a few words the main features of the relationship the physician had with him during examination and interview. This section of the record is called the *Patient Profile*. In addition to a brief personality assessment of the patient, it can contain notes on how he spends his time, his concerns, and his reactions to his life situation, environment, and illness. Other revealing data about the patient, or the physician's response to him, may also be useful. By reading the profile, someone unfamiliar with the patient should rapidly get a picture of him, of how he appeared and behaved at the time of evaluation. Additions to the patient profile or changes in his behavior should be recorded as current observations in the progress notes of the record.

The patient profile can be entered into the record at several points. We prefer to have it at the beginning of the record, after the section on the patient's presenting complaints, because it provides a background view of the patient against which the reader may interpret the recorded data. Alternatively it can be placed just before the physical examination since it represents a transitional point between the historical record and the physician's observations. Again, local conventions and personal preferences should be permitted some flexibility in the organization of the record.

Physical Examination

The physical examination should be recorded in the conventional format found in most textbooks of physical diagnosis. These data are organized primarily by body regions but some observations are related to a specific organ system. The vital signs are recorded first. The conventional brief statement of general observations about the patient has already been recorded in the patient profile.

If a physical examination reveals no abnormalities, the experienced physician creating records for his own use may choose only to state, "All physical findings are within normal limits," after recording the vital signs. Students and house officers are well advised to record their normal findings under specific organ systems and body regions to ensure that the patient has been thoroughly examined, or to note the extent to which each organ system or anatomical area has been examined if circumstances required a limited examination.

Mental Status Examination

A mental status examination is an important part of every physical examination. It can be very brief or quite detailed, depending on the patient, but in every instance the following items should be evaluated: appearance and behavior; speech; mood; thought content; perception; orientation with regard to time, space, and person (or self).

It is obvious that a physician can evaluate many of these items while taking the history and performing the physical examination. Careful observation of the patient from the outset will usually provide most of the data, especially in the areas of appearance, speech, and mood. Patients with blatant disturbances of thought, perception, and orientation may reveal them in the course of the interview. But with many patients, a careful inquiry about their mood, thought content, perception, and orientation is necessary. Mental status is discussed in more detail in Chapter 4. The mental status findings, if not assignable to a problem, should be labeled "Mental Status" and recorded at the end of the physical findings.

It is convenient to leave some space at the end of each section in the Data Base part of the record. As new items of information arise during future contacts with the patient, they can be recorded with the similar information in the appropriate section of the record. Or, if space is not available in the same section of the record, new information may be recorded with the progress notes that follow the sections on identified problems. These entries should be dated and entitled "Additions to data base."

Observations vs. Interpretations

It is mandatory that persons writing in the medical record make clear the distinction between their observations and their interpretations of these observations. Of the two, the objective observations are the more important. The same observation may be interpretable in several ways by different physicians involved in the patient's care, but this is not possible if the primary objective data are not recorded.

Records of Patient Progress

After the record of a new patient has been prepared, all subsequent material entered into the record (progress notes) should be identified by the number and title of the problem to which it is related. Use of the brief problem title makes the record easier to follow for someone seeing it for the first time, especially when the problem list is long. This section of the record should be kept chronologically, with each entry dated and the time of day noted. It is particularly important to enter in these notes pertinent laboratory data, negative and positive, as well as brief summaries or interpretations or radiographic and physiologic studies, even though these may be recorded in more extended form in other sections of the chart. New formulations, established diagnoses, and particularly plans for further study and treatment (all with a brief statement of the rationale involved) are important parts of the chronological follow-up notes. The course of a single problem, and the thought processes of the responsible physician in his efforts to solve that problem, can be followed with ease in such a medical record. This is particularly useful to consultants called to see a patient with whom they are not familiar. Ideally, not a single laboratory or diagnostic procedure should appear in a medical record for which a preceding rationale and subsequent interpretation of the result does not appear in the problem notes. This may help to control the excessive and thoughtless use of these diagnostic aides which is happening in American medicine today.

Weed has proposed that the data about a given problem arising from the patient's own perceptions be categorized as "subjective," and those data which are directly or indirectly observable by the health professional be categorized as "objective." Some difficulties may be encountered in the strict application of this dichotomy. Is the patient's memory of a past medical event a subjective or an objective datum? It may be easier to divide the data into "Historical data" and "Observations." Other titles may be used for these two kinds of information and on occasion intermingling them may improve the clarity of the presentation. Strict separation of the data into categories is not an essential feature of the problem-oriented record. The aim should always be the concise, unambiguous presentation of useful information, while indicating its source. Some variations in style and format are useful in this regard and should be encouraged. Many institutions now employing the P.O.R. have introduced a number of modifications of the basic P.O.R. system of Weed.[5, 6]

The Use of Graphic and Tabular Records

The worn aphorism about the relative value of pictures and words often applies to the medical record. Graphic presentations of numerical data which vary over time in a way that reflects the course of an illness are almost always preferable to a series of verbose notes. Graphic presentations allow the rapid detection and analysis of trends which may be more significant than the absolute levels of certain variables. Discrepant data are more easily detected when in graphic or tabular form. Brief notes can be written at appropriate times on graphs and correlated with the numerical data, but care should be taken not to clutter up an otherwise clear graph.

Graphs

A few general principles are helpful in creating good graphic records. Standard graph paper with squares of about one-half inch can be used for most purposes. It is better than pen-ruled lines on hospital record paper. The crux of the matter lies in selecting the proper dimensions for the axes of the graph. In general, the expected range of the variables plus a little additional space at the end of that range should be laid out on the vertical axis. It is not necessary to start the graph at zero unless the variable can be expected to approach this value. Intervals which are multiples or fractions of 1, 2, 5, 10, 20, 50, 100, etc., are usually easily interpreted. Choice of appropriate time intervals along the base axis is equally important. This choice depends on the expected frequency of observations or the rate at which the variables can be expected to change. A little thought about these questions will also help decide whether the proposed frequency of observation is excessive, adequate, or insufficient before the management of a patient's problem has progressed very far. Do not try to plot more than the minimal significant data. Choose data that are likely to show some important direct or inverse correlation for the same graph. Colored pens or pencils are essential in keeping lines separated if they come close together. Crossing of lines should be avoided by proper choice of vertical axis dimensions and by plotting the several variables one above the other with sufficient space in between. The axes and the units involved should be clearly labeled.

It is advantageous to work out blank graph forms with the axes drawn in, numbered, and labeled for some of the common medical and surgical problems in which graphs are particularly useful. Master sheets reflecting the record needs of problems like diabetic acidosis, gastrointestinal bleeding, and respiratory failure can be drawn up in advance and reproduced for use in records by a copying machine. The master sheets are then easily revised as experience or the availability of new knowledge dictates.

Tabular Records

Tabular recording of data has many of the same advantages of graphs, and most of the general rules of graphic presentation also apply to constructing good tables. Tables are best adapted to record data that must be summarized in verbal form, or mixed verbal and numerical data. Therapy is particularly well summarized in tables. In medical problems such as the management of cardiac arrhythmias, fluid and electrolyte balance in intestinal obstruction, dialysis, and tumor chemotherapy it may be useful to have a tabular display of data. Tables should not be crowded, nor should they contain redundant data or data that is not essential. Columns should be used for the observations and should be clearly labeled with units indicated. The rows of a table are used for observations at a given time. Timing of observations can be predetermined at the time of initial management planning. This is again strongly recommended as an aid to rational, efficient, and comprehensive treatment and documentation of a medical or surgical problem.

We wish to stress the value of graphic and tabular records in patient management, provided that critical data are chosen for display and then reviewed regularly for departure from expected trends, inconsistencies, errors, and warning signs that other problems may be appearing. Physicians regularly use charts of the patient's vital signs. Graphic and tabular data are a major but quite similar extension of this already familiar record device.

Minimum Requirements of a Problem-Oriented Record

We have pointed out that some variations of the format have been developed and are in use in major institutions. What features are essential if the record is to keep its problem orientation? It seems to us that there are three such criteria:

1. The record is introduced by a Master Problem List that identifies to the best of the physician's ability the patient's past and present problems of medical significance. This list must be comprehensive.
2. The record must integrate relevant data about each problem with an evaluation of its nature and importance and plans for its management.
3. The record must reflect the process of patient care as well as

the data upon which that care is based. The rationale for interpretations of the data and therapeutic decisions must appear.

3 A BRIEF GUIDE TO THE P.O.R.*

We present below a brief guide to the P.O.R. as it is now employed in our institution, along with an example of a record constructed in both the conventional and the problem-oriented format. This patient record in P.O.R. format is somewhat modified from the structure suggested by Weed as the ultimate form of P.O.R. We feel, however, that it still serves the main purpose of the P.O.R. The same record is again presented in Chapter 11 in relation to computer-based record-keeping and other advanced data-handling technologies. There, the data are further broken down, assigned to identified problems, and recorded in an integrated form by problems. The reader may wish to compare these two problem-oriented records.

CONTENT OF THE DATA BASE

I. Patient's Complaints

II. Patient Profile

Description of the patient, how he spends an average day, and relevant social data

III. Present Illness or Illnesses

A. Includes chief complaints and current problems

B. Each problem considered and recorded separately

C. Historical data, recorded under each titled problem in four categories

1. Symptomatic (SX)—symptoms, i.e. information obtained through the patient's perceptions.

* The authors are grateful to Dr. Paul Hollister, Instructor in Medicine, Michigan State University College of Human Medicine, for his help in developing this material and evaluating its use by students and house officers.

2. Objective (OBJ)—documented post observational data, i.e. old record data such as physical findings, laboratory and x-ray data, data from surgery and biopsies
3. Treatment (RX)—medications, diet, physical therapy, etc.
4. Significant Negatives (NEG)—pertinent data related to titled problems

IV. Past History, Family History, and Review of Systems
V. Present Physical Examination
VI. Initial Diagnostic Studies
- A. CBC
- B. Urinalysis
- C. VDRL
- D. Chest x-ray
- E. EKG when indicated

DEVELOPMENT OF THE MASTER PROBLEM LIST

This is a numbered list of all significant problems, present and past, resolved and unresolved, medical, psychiatric, and social. This list is the first page of the P.O.R., although it can be constructed only after the data base is available.

Each problem is listed at a level of refinement that is known and will fall into one of four categories. (No diagnostic guesses!):

1. Etiologic Diagnosis, e.g. atherosclerotic heart disease.
2. Physiological Finding, e.g. congestive heart failure.
3. Symptom or Physical Finding, e.g. shortness of breath or tachypnea.
4. Abnormal Laboratory Finding, e.g. abnormal EKG.

There are several conventions in keeping the Master Problem List:

1.) If a numbered diagnosis has several manifestations, these are included with the diagnosis, for example:

1) Cirrhosis
   Jaundice
2) Ascites (minimal)

2.) If one of these manifestations is or becomes therapeutically significant, requiring management, it is entered as a separate problem, and indicated as secondary to a numbered diagnosis:

1) Cirrhosis
Jaundice
2) Ascites—secondary to problem 1.

3.) When a problem is clarified, the original list is modified with the date:

5) Sore throat $\underrightarrow{6/16/69}$ Streptococcal pharyngitis.
9) Shortness of breath $\underrightarrow{6/21/69}$ Congestive heart failure.

4.) Problems are recorded in active or inactive columns as appropriate:

Cholecystectomy 10 years before is inactive.

5.) When a problem is resolved, a dated arrow is again used:

2) Pneumococcal pneumonia $\underrightarrow{6/30/69}$ Resolved.

6.) If the etiology of a symptom or physiological finding is not definitely known, then the statement "etiology unknown" follows the numbered problem:

2) Vertigo, etiology unknown. (No "probable," "question of" or "rule-outs" belong in the problem list.)

FORMULATION OF INITIAL PLAN

This section of the record concludes the basic record of the patient, and precedes the progress notes. For each numbered active problem, there is a corresponding numbered and titled plan with three entries:

1.) Data Collection, e.g. diagnostic studies needed.
2.) Treatment, e.g. medications, procedures.
3.) Patient Education—a brief statement of what the patient is told about the diagnosis and plan of management.

Under each numbered undiagnosed problem is included the differential diagnosis of that problem with a separate plan for each possibility, as above, for example:

1) Coin Lesion of Lung by X-ray
   - Carcinoma?
     - Tomograms
     - Sputum for cytology
     - Bronchoscopy
   - Tuberculosis?
     - PPD Test
     - Sputum studies acid—fast bacilli
     - Bronchial washings culture
   - Bacterial pneumonia?
     - Sputum cultures

PREPARATION OF PROGRESS NOTES

Significant information should be incorporated into the progress notes in the problem-oriented format. This includes data from the patient, laboratory, x-ray, consultations, and conferences.

Notes are written separately for each problem and are numbered and titled according to the master problem list. For each problem any or all of the following elements are entered:

1.) Symptomatic (SX.)
2.) Objective (OBJ.)
3.) Assessment (ASSES.)
4.) Immediate Plan (PLAN.)

When new problems arise, they are numbered and added to the problem list with the date of the progress note to which they refer.

PROBLEM-ORIENTED TABULAR RECORDS

I. Objectives
   - A. Concise and accurate record of serially obtained data in both acute and chronic disorders
   - B. Selection and organization of pertinent observations followed for specific problems
   - C. Clarity of interrelationships of multiple, changing observations and treatment over a period of time

D. Ease of interpretation of interrelated and changing variables
E. Temporal correlation of observed changes due to, or coincident with, treatment

II. Indications
A. Any clinical condition requiring repetitive, *serial data analysis* over a period of time
B. Any clinical problem involving expected *changes in several observations* over a period of time
C. Any clinical condition with *multiple problems* and hence multiple observations, i.e. more than one organ system involved
D. Any condition requiring *multiple treatments* simultaneously or sequentially administered
E. *Summaries of old records* with repetitive data and treatments

III. Construction
A. Choice of variables

For every problem where the treatment may be changed, variables for evaluation of results should be selected. The following are illustrative examples:

1. "Organ failure" observations

In a case of liver failure one might follow the patient's weight, liver size, abdominal girth, alcohol intake, mental functions, asterixis, bilirubin, alkaline phosphatase, SGOT, serum albumin, Na^+ and K^+, diuretic therapy, diet, and protein intake.

2. "Major abnormality" observations

If a major complaint or finding in the patient with liver failure was ascites, observations of body weight, urine volume, and diuretic therapy would be selected.

3. Urine volume and fluid balance

These observations are frequently important in many clinical problems and require that serial data be obtained.

4. Medications, particularly if more than one drug is given sequentially or concurrently
   In a case of congestive heart failure, one might tabulate digoxin, mercuhydrin, diuril, aldactone, diet, Na^+ intake, and water intake.
5. Potential changes of clinical course (Complications)
   In a case of chronic lymphocytic leukemia, tabulation of the hematocrit, Coomb's test, and reticulocyte count might be obtained anticipating the onset of hemolysis.

B. Choice of time coordinate. Frequency of measurements or observations and their recording is determined by the expected rate of change or frequency of potential changes. For example, in cases of rheumatoid arthritis, the time scale is months-years, in diabetic acidosis, hours, and in cardiac arrhythmia, it is minutes-days.

REFERENCES

1. Weed, L. L., "Medical Records That Guide and Teach," *New England Journal of Medicine*, 278:593, 1967, and 278:652, 1967.
2. Weed, L. L., "New Approach to Medical Teaching," *Resident Physician*, 13:77, 1967.
3. Weed, L. L., *Medical Records, Medical Education and Patient Care, The Problem-Oriented Record as a Basic Tool*. Cleveland: The Press of Case Western Reserve University, 1969.
4. Bjorn, J. C., and H. D. Cross, *The Problem Oriented Private Practice of Medicine, A System for Comprehensive Health Care*. Chicago: Modern Hospital Press, 1970.
5. Ways, P. O., T. Baker, P. Finkelstein, N. Fiel, and J. W. Jones. "The Problem Oriented Record (A Self-Instructional Unit)." Published by College of Human Medicine, Michigan State University, East Lansing, 1969.
6. Voytovich, A. "Using the Problem Oriented Medical Record (The Weed System)." Published by Cleveland Metropolitan General Hospital, Cleveland, 1970.

EXAMPLES OF CLINICAL RECORDS

On the pages following will be found an example of the conventional record format and the problem-oriented format for a single episode of illness. The same information is not presented in both.

MICHIGAN STATE UNIVERSITY HEALTH CENTER
East Lansing, Michigan 48823
CLINICAL RECORD (CONVENTIONAL FORMAT)

Date & Time | Patient Name: Miss Mary Blank | Unit Record No. 16711

CHIEF COMPLAINT: "My menstrual periods are too heavy."

1/10/72 9 a.m. PRESENT ILLNESS: This 42 year old single woman noticed increasingly heavy menstrual flow about 8 months ago. Since then periods have lasted 7 to 9 days during which she daily soaked through several standard pads. The periods were normally timed, without discomfort or other notable symptoms.

Three months ago, a normally timed period started that lasted 12 days. She passed clots on the second, third, and fourth days, which she spent in bed. Since this period, she has had intermittent vaginal bleeding, every 3 to 5 days, varying in amount from slight spotting to enough to require 2 to 3 pads daily and lasting a day or two at a time. She thinks she has had one normally timed period, starting about December 5, 1971. This was also heavy and prolonged. She did not seek medical care because she felt this problem was due to "change of life."

In spite of the excessive menstrual bleeding, she felt quite well until about 4 months ago when she began to experience increasing fatigue, decreased exercise tolerance, and weight loss of about 14 lbs. She feels she has also become increasingly pale and has taken a proprietary iron tablet twice daily for several months. She feels her appetite has increased if it has changed at all and she has eaten regularly. She has not felt tremulous or noted heat intolerance. Nor has she noted excessive thirst or increased urine volume, although she has habitually urinated frequently.

Two days ago, in the late afternoon, she began to feel much worse with onset of nausea, anorexia, and greatly increased weakness. She has been somewhat somnolent since. She was brought to the hospital by a friend who called at her apartment to take her to work and found her still in bed.

PAST HISTORY: She has enjoyed good health in general, except for intermittent joint swelling, pain, and stiffness in the hands, wrists, and shoulders, as well as occasionally in other joints for the past six years. This was diagnosed as rheumatoid arthritis at the University of Michigan Clinics in 1968. She has had little joint deformity but intermittently takes as many as 12 aspirin tablets a day for pain. She has been taking aspirin in doses of 6 to 12 tablets a day for the last 2 months. Occasionally, she takes a proprietary "extra strength" product, the name of which she cannot recall now.

She had measles, mumps, chicken pox, and acute tonsillitis as a child. Her only surgical operation was a tonsillectomy at age 9 which was uneventful. She has not had other hemorrhagic manifestations in the past or with the present illness.

Prepared by: ______________________ Staff title/Student status ______________________

MICHIGAN STATE UNIVERSITY HEALTH CENTER
East Lansing, Michigan 48823
CLINICAL RECORD (CONVENTIONAL FORMAT)

Date & Time | Patient Name: Miss Mary Blank | Unit Record No. 16711

FAMILY HISTORY: The patient has never married. She was the only child of parents both now deceased. Her father died in 1950 at age 43 of a heart attack. Her mother died in November 1969 of metastatic carcinoma of the colon at age 61. Miss Blank lived with her mother prior to her death. Her parents were both of English origin. A paternal aunt, age about 50, has diabetes. She thinks her paternal grandmother also had diabetes. Otherwise there is no history of familial diseases, including hemorrhagic disorders or anemia.

SOCIAL HISTORY: Miss Blank was born on January 5, 1930, on a farm south of Lansing, Michigan, and grew up there. After high school, she studied fine arts at Michigan State University for two years. She commuted from home and earned most of her expenses as a stenographer. After her father's death, she stopped attending college, moved to Lansing with her mother, and began to work as a secretary in a legal office. She describes her mother as a dependent, inadequate person who was recurrently depressed after her father's death. She speaks without overt resentment of "having devoted my entire life to mother." She describes herself as a lonely, isolated person with few friends, mixture of sadness, relief, and guilt over her sense of relief following her mother's death. She has had recurrent insomnia, feelings of sadness, and hopelessness; she cried daily for the month after her mother died. She has felt somewhat better from this point of view in the last few months. She still has occasional periods of sadness and crying. She has been able to keep up with her demanding position of office manager in the legal office where she has worked for over 20 years.

REVIEW OF SYSTEMS: Only the following significant data were obtained:

Allergies: None known.

Eyes: She has not noted any vision changes; she wears glasses.

Mouth: She has lost both lower right molar teeth and they are unreplaced.

Neck: She has never had a goiter or any other evidence of thyroid disease; her voice is unchanged.

Skin: She has had no evidence of excessive bruising or petechial hemorrhages. She has had no pigmentary changes, changes in their distribution, or other characteristics.

G.U.: (In addition to PI) She has had no pregnancies.

Prepared by: ____________________ Staff title/Student status ____________________

MICHIGAN STATE UNIVERSITY HEALTH CENTER
East Lansing, Michigan 48823
CLINICAL RECORD (CONVENTIONAL FORMAT)

Date & Time

Patient Name: Miss Mary Blank Unit Record No. 16711

CNS: During the last 5 years, she has had headaches 1 to 3 times weekly, characterized by a feeling of tightness in the back of her head and neck and head pain which radiates forward bilaterally from this region. She has no visual or other aura or related phenomena. The headaches are precipatated by fatigue, excessive work stress, and frustration. They are promptly relieved by rest and aspirin.

Habits: Does not drink or smoke, and has not in the past. Takes no drugs regularly except aspirin and related products. Describes her diet as well balanced with meals precisely timed. Weight has averaged 124 lbs. over past 10 years varying only a few pounds. Highest weight, 130 in 1952.

PHYSICAL EXAMINATION: Pulse 95 BPM: Temp. 38 C p.o.; Resp. 19/min.; BP 108/70 Right arm reclining; Ht. 66"; Wt. 110 lbs. The patient is a rather tall, thin, pale woman who looks somewhat older than her stated age. She looks both chronically and acutely ill. She responds precisely to all questions, and she speaks somewhat slowly, without apparent emotion. She interacts minimally on interview and examination.

Skin: Normal except for some loss of turgor suggesting dehydration.

Head: Eyes are normal except for a moderate narrowing of the arteries and some increased tortuosity.

Ears, Nose, Throat: Normal. Mouth: The tongue is heavily coated. The mucosae appear moderately dehydrated and pale. Lower right molar teeth missing. The remaining teeth are in good repair, but the gingivae appear red, slightly swollen, and retracted around the canine and lateral incisors in the lower jaw.

Neck: The thyroid gland is palpable, smooth, and normal in size. The neck normal.

Lymphatic System: A soft 1/2 cm. node is palpable high in the left axilla. No other notable glands.

Chest: Normal configuration. Respiration is somewhat deeper than normal and slightly accelerated.

Lungs: Clear in all areas.

Heart: Normal rhythm. Tachycardia is persistent. Heart size, shape, and sounds are normal.

Peripheral Vessels: Brachial arteries feel normal. All pulses normally palpable. Veins and venous pressure appear to be normal. No edema.

Prepared by: ______________________ ______________________
Staff title/Student status

MICHIGAN STATE UNIVERSITY HEALTH CENTER
East Lansing, Michigan 48823
CLINICAL RECORD (CONVENTIONAL FORMAT)

Date & Time | Patient Name: Miss Mary Blank | Unit Record No. 16711

Breasts: Small, showing evidence of recent weight loss. No abnormalities.

Abdomen: There is slight mid-abdominal distension and tympany. No organs or masses are palpable. There is distinct tenderness and some guarding on deep suprapubic palpation. The CVA are negative.

Pelvic Examination: The external genitalia are normal. The introitus is virginal and speculum and manual examination were unsatisfactory. The vaginal mucosa appears normal as does the cervix. There was no bleeding. There was tenderness anteriorly on palpation. The uterus was thought to be 3 to 4 times normal size and somewhat irregular in contour.

Rectal Examination: Confirms above findings. There are no rectal abnormalities.

Extremities: The proximal interphalangeal joints of both hands show thickening, slight limitation of motion on flexion with tapering of the fingers. The skin of the fingers is smooth but thin and supple. The right wrist is also affected. The remaining joints appear normal and exhibit normal mobility.

Neurological: Within normal limits. There is no tremor.

Mental Status: Appearance and behavior: quiet, reserved, pale, colorless; responds slowly, looks sad, never smiles. Speech: soft voice; clear but brief answers; never elaborates unless encouraged. Mood: looks depressed. Admits to feeling "blue." States this has improved recently. Thought content: still grieving for her mother. No suicidal ideas. No evidence of psychotic thought disorder. Orientation: clear.

LABORATORY FINDINGS

Hematology: Hematocrit 30%, Hgb. 8.8 gm.%; WBC 11,000/cu. mm. Differential count: Polys. 60%, Band forms 4%, Eosinophils 1%, Basophils 0%, Monocytes 7%, Lymphocytes 28%. The red cells show hypochromia, anisocytosis, microcytosis, and polychromasia. The leukocytes are normal in appearance. Platelets are present in normal numbers and appear normal.

Urinalysis: pH 5.0, specific gravity 1.035, cloudy, dark amber. Glucose 2+, Acetone 2+, protein Tr, Micro: Rare WBC. Gram stain - few gram neg. rods.

Prepared by: ____________________ Staff title/Student status ____________________

MICHIGAN STATE UNIVERSITY HEALTH CENTER
East Lansing, Michigan 48823

CLINICAL RECORD (CONVENTIONAL FORMAT)

Date & Time

Patient Name: Miss Mary Blank Unit Record No. 16711

IMPRESSIONS:

1. Uterine bleeding, cause unknown, probably due to intrauterine pathology.
2. ?Diabetes mellitus.
3. Rheumatoid Arthritis.
4. Depression.
5. Anemia, probably iron deficiency due to blood loss.

DIAGNOSTIC AND THERAPEUTIC PLAN:

1. Gyn consultation for exam under anesthesia, pap smears, and possible biopsy or D & C.
2. Blood sugar, BUN, and electrolyte determinations stat.
3. Bone marrow examination for iron stores. If low, administer ferrous sulphate in increasing doses, starting with 0.2 gm. p.o. with largest meal. Measure prothrombin concentration, stools for blood.
4. Request information from University of Michigan Arthritis Clinic. No medication for present.
5. Patient will be evaluated on medical psychiatric rounds tomorrow.

1/11/72 11:00 a.m.

PROGRESS NOTES

The patient feels a little better today. She has stopped bleeding. She is more communicative, and has added the information that she has been taking some "nerve pills" obtained from a friend. We are attempting to find out what these are.

She is not bleeding at present. The blood glucose yesterday was 320 mg.%, the BUN 25 mg.%, the CO_2 20mM/L, Na+ 135, K+5 and Cl^- 100 m Eq/L. She is diabetic. She was placed on a regimen of 6 hour blocks of feeding and insulin. She is receiving 10 u. regular insulin and 500 calories per block. On this program, her blood sugar was 150 mg.% at 2:00 p.m. today and her urine sugar negative.

She also got 2,000 cc. of normal saline IV yesterday and was given orange juice as part of her oral feedings. Since she was not in severe acidosis, it seems likely that the nerve pills were causing her mildly obtunded state.

The bone marrow examination has not yet been done. The reticulocyte count is 5% and the red cell indices show hypochromia and microcytosis of mild degree.

John Black, M.D. Medical Intern

Prepared by: Staff title/Student status

MICHIGAN STATE UNIVERSITY HEALTH CENTER
East Lansing, Michigan 48823

CLINICAL RECORD (CONVENTIONAL FORMAT)

Date & Time | Patient Name: Miss Mary Blank | Unit Record No. 16711

1/11/72 4 p.m. Dr. Enelow and Dr. Swisher saw this patient in medical-psychiatric conference. It was felt that the diagnosis was more specifically adjustment reaction of adult life and that she was going through a normal grief response following her mother's death. The steady improvement and her ability to talk about her grief were felt to indicate a good prognosis.

She also has fears about having cancer "like mother," which was brought out at the conference interview. At present, we cannot reassure her about this possibility. We have told her that there are several other more likely possibilities to account for her bleeding and that we will know more about this problem soon after she is seen by Dr. Regis of the Gyn service.

We will give her psychologically supportive care on the medical service, encouraging her to discuss her feelings about her medical problem and life situation. Miss Jones of Social Service will also see her daily, talk with her and assist her with several problems, including renewal of her lease, deciding about sharing apartment, and obtaining a sick leave. Antidepressant drug therapy is not indicated, in view of the normal progression of her grief reaction.

R. J. Peel, M.D. — Medical Resident

Prepared by: — Staff title/Student status

MICHIGAN STATE UNIVERSITY HEALTH CENTER
East Lansing, Michigan 48823

NAME Miss Mary Blank UNIT RECORD NO. 16711

MASTER PROBLEM LIST

PROB #	DATE ONSET	ACTIVE PROBLEM	RESOLVED PROBLEM	DATE RESOL.
1	1/10/72	Uterine Bleeding Etiology Unknown		
2	1/10/72	Weight Loss 1/11/72 Diabetes Mellitus		
3	1/10/72	Arthritis Etiology Unknown		
4	1/10/72	Depression 1/11/72 Adjustment reaction of adult life (grief reaction)		
5	1/10/72	Anemia, Secondary to problem 1		

MICHIGAN STATE UNIVERSITY HEALTH CENTER
East Lansing, Michigan 48823

CLINICAL RECORD (PROBLEM-ORIENTED FORMAT)

Date & Time | Patient Name: Miss Mary Blank | Unit Record No. 16711

DATA BASE

1/10/72 9 a.m. PATIENT'S COMPLAINT: "My menstrual periods are too heavy."

PATIENT PROFILE: This patient is a 42 year old single white woman, a law office secretary, who was brought to the hospital by a friend who called for her this morning to take her to work and found her still in bed. The patient has no voluntary complaints, but on questioning first states that "my menstrual periods are too heavy," and also indicates that she is weak and losing weight. She is reserved and quiet and seems sad.

PROBLEM #1 Vaginal bleeding: This woman noticed increasingly heavy menstrual flow about 8 months ago. Periods have lasted 7 to 9 days during which she daily soaked through several standard pads. The periods were normally timed, without discomfort or other notable symptoms.

Three months ago, a normally timed period started and lasted 12 days. She passed clots on the second, third, and fourth days which she spent in bed. Since this period, she has had intermittent vaginal bleeding, every 3 to 5 days, varying in amount from slight spotting to enough to require 2 to 3 pads daily, lasting a day or two at a time. She thinks she has had one normally timed period, starting about December 5, 1971. This was also heavy and prolonged. She did not seek medical care because she felt this problem was due to "change of life." She has had no pregnancies.

Two days ago, in the late afternoon, she began to feel much worse with onset of nausea, anorexia, and greatly increased weakness. She has been somewhat somnolent since.

PROBLEM #2 Weight loss: She felt quite well until about 4 months ago, when she began to experience increasing fatigue, decreased exercise tolerance, and weight loss of about 14 pounds. She feels her appetite has increased if anything and she has eaten regularly. She has not felt tremulous or noted heat intolerance. Neither has she noted excessive thirst or increased urine volume, although she habitually urinated frequently. A paternal aunt, age 50, has diabetes. She thinks her paternal grandmother also had diabetes.

She describes her diet as well balanced with meals precisely timed. Weight has averaged 124 lbs. over past 10 years varying only a few pounds. Highest weight 130 in 1952.

She has not noted vision changed. She has never had a goiter or any other evidence of thyroid disease; her voice is unchanged.

PROBLEM #3 Arthritis: She has had intermittent joint swelling, pain and stiffness in the hands, wrists, and shoulders, as well as occasionally in other joints for the past six years. She has had little joint deformity.

Prepared by: ____________________ Staff title/Student status ____________________

MICHIGAN STATE UNIVERSITY HEALTH CENTER
East Lansing, Michigan 48823

CLINICAL RECORD (PROBLEM-ORIENTED FORMAT)

Date & Time | Patient Name: Miss Mary Blank | Unit Record No. 16711

This was diagnosed as rheumatoid arthritis at the University of Michigan Clinics in 1968. Intermittently she takes as many as 12 aspirin tablets a day for pain. For the last 2 months she has been taking aspirin in doses of 6 to 12 tablets a day. Occasionally, she takes a proprietary "extra strength" product, the name of which she cannot recall now.

PROBLEM #4 Depression: This woman lived with her mother who died of metastatic carcinoma of the colon in November 1969 at age 61. She feels a mixture of sadness, relief, and guilt over her sense of relief following her mother's death. She has had recurrent insomnia, feelings of sadness and hopelessness, and cried daily for the month after her mother died.

She has felt somewhat better from this point of view in the last few months. She still has occasional periods of sadness and crying. She has been able to keep up with her demanding position as office manager in the legal office where she has worked for over 20 years.

During the last 5 years, she has had headaches 1 to 3 times weekly characterized by a feeling of tightness in the back of her head and neck and head pain which radiates forward bilaterally from this region. She has no visual or other aura or related phenomena. The headaches are precipatated by fatigue, excessive work stress, and frustration. They are promptly relieved by rest and aspirin.

PROBLEM #5 Anemia: She has had excessive blood loss as noted in problem #1. She feels she has become increasingly pale, and she has taken a proprietary iron tablet twice daily for several months. She has not been known to be anemic in the past and there is no familial history of anemia.

PAST MEDICAL HISTORY: She had measles, mumps, chicken pox, and acute tonsillitis as a child. Her only surgical operation was a tonsillectomy at age 9 which was uneventful. She has not had other hemorrhagic manifestations in the past or with the present illness.

FAMILY HISTORY: The patient has never married. She was the only child; both of her parents are now deceased. Her father died in 1950 at age 43 of a heart attack. Her mother died in November 1969 of metastatic carcinoma of the colon at age 61. Miss Blank lived with her mother prior to her death. Her parents were both of English origin. A paternal aunt, age about 50, has diabetes. She thinks her paternal grandmother also had diabetes. Otherwise there is no history of familial diseases, including hemorrhagic disorders or anemia.

Prepared by: ______________ Staff title/Student status ______________

MICHIGAN STATE UNIVERSITY HEALTH CENTER
East Lansing, Michigan 48823

CLINICAL RECORD (PROBLEM-ORIENTED FORMAT)

Date & Time | Patient Name: Miss Mary Blank | Unit Record No. 16711

SOCIAL HISTORY: Miss Blank was born on January 5, 1930, on a farm south of Lansing, Michigan, and grew up there. After high school, she studied fine arts at Michigan State University for two years. She commuted from home and earned most of her expenses as a stenographer. After her father's death, she stopped attending college, moved to Lansing with her mother and began to work as a secretary in a legal office. She describes her mother as a dependent, inadequate person who was recurrently depressed after her father's death. She speaks without overt resentment of "having devoted my entire life to mother." She describes herself as a lonely, isolated person with few friends.

REVIEW OF SYSTEMS: Only the following significant data were obtained:

Allergies: None known.

Eyes: She has not noted any vision changes; she wears glasses.

Mouth: She has lost both lower right molar teeth and they are unreplaced.

Neck: She has never had a goiter or any other evidence of thyroid disease; her voice is unchanged.

Skin: She has had no evidence of excessive bruising or petechial hemorrhages. She has had no pigmentary changes, changes in hair distribution, or other characteristics.

G.U.: (In addition to PI) She has had no pregnancies.

CNS: During the last 5 years, she has had headaches 1 to 3 times weekly characterized by a feeling of tightness in the back of her head and neck and head pain which radiates forward bilaterally from this region. She has no visual or other aura or related phenomena. The headaches are precipitated by fatigue, excessive work stress, and frustration. They are promptly relieved by rest and aspirin.

Habits: Does not drink or smoke, and has not in the past. Takes no drugs regularly except aspirin and related products. Describes her diet as well balanced with meals precisely timed. Weight has averaged 124 lbs. over past 10 years varying only a few pounds. Highest weight, 130 in 1952.

PHYSICAL EXAMINATION: Pulse 95 BPM; Temp. 38°C p.o.; Resp. 19/min.; BP 108/70 Right arm reclining; Ht. 66"; Wt. 110 lbs. The patient is a rather tall, thin, pale woman who looks somewhat older than her stated age. She looks both chronically and

Prepared by: ______________________ Staff title/Student status ______________________

CLINICAL RECORD (PROBLEM-ORIENTED FORMAT)

Date & Time Patient Name: Miss Mary Blank Unit Record No. 16711

acutely ill. She responds precisely to all questions, but somewhat slowly, without apparent emotion. She interacts minimally on interview and examination.

Skin: Normal except for some loss of turgor suggesting dehydration.

Head: Eyes are normal except for a moderate narrowing of the arteries and some increased tortuosity.

Ears, Nose, Throat: Normal. Mouth: The tongue is heavily coated. The mucosae appear moderately dehydrated and pale. Lower right molar teeth missing. The remaining teeth are in good repair but the gingivae appear red, slightly swollen, and retracted around the canine and lateral incisors in the lower jaw.

Neck: The thyroid gland is palpable, smooth, and normal in size. The neck is normal.

Lymphatic System: A soft 1/2 cm. node is palpable high in the left axilla. No other notable glands.

Chest: Normal configuration. Respiration is somewhat deeper than normal and slightly accelerated.

Lungs: Clear in all areas.

Heart: Normal rhythm. Tachycardia is persistent. Heart size, shape, and sounds are normal.

Peripheral Vessels: Brachial arteries feel normal. All pulses normally palpable. Veins and venous pressure appear to be normal. No edema.

Breasts: Small, showing evidence of recent weight loss. No abnormalities.

Abdomen: There is slight mid-abdominal distension and tympany. No organs or masses are palpable. There is distinct tenderness and some guarding on deep suprapubic palpation. The CVA are negative.

Pelvic Examination: The external genitalia are normal. The introitus is virginal and speculum and manual examination were unsatisfactory. The vaginal mucosa appears normal as does the cervix. There was no bleeding. There was tenderness anteriorly on palpation. The uterus was thought to be 3 to 4 times normal size and somewhat irregular in contour.

Prepared by: ______________________ Staff title/Student status

MICHIGAN STATE UNIVERSITY HEALTH CENTER
East Lansing, Michigan 48823

CLINICAL RECORD (PROBLEM-ORIENTED FORMAT)

Date & Time | Patient Name: Miss Mary Blank | Unit Record No. 16711

Rectal Examination: Confirms above findings. There are no rectal abnormalities.

Extremities: The proximal interphalangeal joints of both hands show thickening, slight limitation of motion on flexion with tapering of the fingers. The skin of the fingers is smooth, but thin and supple. The right wrist is also affected. The remaining joints appear normal and exhibit normal mobility.

Neurological: Within normal limits. There is no tremor.

Mental Status: Appearance and behavior - quiet, reserved, pale, colorless, responds slowly, looks sad, never smiles. Speech - soft voice; clear but brief answers; never elaborates unless encouraged. Mood - looks depressed. Admits to feeling "blue." States this has improved recently. Thought content - still grieving for her mother. No suicidal ideas. No evidence of psychotic thought disorder. Orientation - clear.

INITIAL LABORATORY FINDINGS:

Hematology: Hematocrit 30%, Hgb. 8.8 gm.%; WBC 11,000/cu. mm., Differential count: Polys. 60%, Band forms 4%, Eosinophils 1%, Basophils 0%, Monocytes 7%, Lymphocytes 28%. The red cells show hypochromia, anisocytosis, microcytosis, and polychromasia. The leukocytes are normal in appearance. Platelets are present in normal numbers and appear normal.

Urinalysis: pH 5.0, specific gravity 1.035, cloudy, dark amber. Glucose 2+, Acetone 2+, protein Tr, Micro - rare WBC. Gram stain - few gram neg. rods.

INITIAL PLAN

PROBLEM #1 Uterine Bleeding

Formulation: The source of the vaginal bleeding appears to be the uterus. The uterine enlargement suggests the presence of a tumor. Distinction between a benign tumor and an endometrial cancer cannot be made on the basis of available data. It is possible, but unlikely, that she has a bleeding diathesis on the basis of the aspirin she has taken. There is no evidence of a generalized hemorrhagic disorder.

Plan: Diagnostic - Gyn consultation for exam under anesthesia, pap smears, and possibly biopsy or D & C. (Dr. Regis)

Prepared by: | Staff title/Student status

MICHIGAN STATE UNIVERSITY HEALTH CENTER
East Lansing, Michigan 48823

CLINICAL RECORD (PROBLEM-ORIENTED FORMAT)

Date & Time

Patient Name: Miss Mary Blank Unit Record No. 16711

Therapeutic - none needed at present.

The diagnostic plan has been discussed with the patient but the differential diagnosis has not been presented to her as yet. The patient agrees to this plan.

PROBLEM #2 Weight Loss

Formulation: The weight loss could be compatible with a malignant uterine tumor, although there is no evidence of metastasis or extension. The glycosuria raises the possibility of diabetes, although she is not in apparent acidosis. Hyperthyroidism or other metabolic or gastrointestinal causes of weight loss seem unlikely.

Plan: Diagnostic - Blood sugar, BUN, and electrolyte determinations stat.
Therapeutic - Start IV fluids and await results above.
Discussion with the patient deferred.

PROBLEM #3 Arthritis

Formulation: Probably rheumatoid disease, with little evidence of activity at the present. Osteoarthritis should be considered.

Plan: Diagnostic - Request information from University of Michigan Arthritis Clinic.
Therapeutic - No medication for present.
Discussion with the patient deferred.

PROBLEM #4 Depression

Formulation: This woman probably has a reactive or situational depression following the death of her mother. She has historical evidence of tension headaches. Her social background suggests a high level of isolation, but she has functioned well in her job, without decompensation. A psychotic depression should be considered.

Plan: Diagnostic - Patient will be evaluated on medical psychiatric rounds tomorrow.
Therapeutic - Dependent upon consultant's recommendation. We will not give her any anti-depressant drugs at present. I discussed the patient's feelings of sadness with her during the interview and suggested to her that she was abnormally depressed. She accepted this formulation and agreed to be seen on rounds tomorrow. She knows who will be in the group and what the procedure will be.

Prepared by: Staff title/Student status

MICHIGAN STATE UNIVERSITY HEALTH CENTER
East Lansing, Michigan 48823

CLINICAL RECORD (PROBLEM-ORIENTED FORMAT)

Date & Time | Patient Name: Miss Mary Blank | Unit Record No. 16711

PROBLEM #5 Anemia

Formulation: The blood picture appears to be that of iron deficiency anemia, probably due to uterine blood loss. There is no evidence of a primary blood dyscrasia, nor of metastatic tumor in bone marrow, but a hypo regenerative anemia secondary to tumor should be considered. Megaloblastic and nutritional anemias seem unlikely.

Plan: Diagnostic - Reticulocyte count, red cell indices. Bone marrow examination for iron stores. Stools for blood.
Therapeutic - If low iron stores, administer ferrous sulphate in increasing doses, starting with 0.2 gm. p.o. with largest meal.
Discussion with patient deferred.

PROGRESS NOTES:

1/11/72 11:00 a.m.

PROBLEM #1 Uterine bleeding: She is not bleeding at present.

PROBLEM #4 Depression: The patient feels a little better today. She is more communicative, and has added the information that she has been taking some "nerve pills" obtained from a friend. We are attempting to find out what these are.

PROBLEM #2 Entitled Diabetes Mellitus: The blood glucose yesterday was 320 mg.% - the BUN 25 mg.%, the CO_2 20 mM/L, Na^+ 135, K^+5 and Cl^- 100 m Eq/L. She is diabetic. She was placed on a regimen of 6 hour blocks of feeding and insulin. She received 10 u. regular insulin and 500 calories per block. On this program, her blood sugar was 150 mg.% at 2:00 p.m. today and her urine sugar negative. She also got 2,000 cc. of normal saline IV yesterday and was given orange juice as part of her oral feedings.

Assessment: Since she was not in severe acidosis, it seems likely that the nerve pills were causing her mildly obtunded state.

Plan: We will carry her on 6 hour program for another day. Since there is no evidence of infection at present, she will be shifted to a single dose of insulin and a program of regulation begun. She will be gotten out of bed today.
Insulin reduced to 6 U. per block today. Will transfer to P2I insulin tomorrow.

PROBLEM #5 Anemia: The bone marrow examination has not yet been done. The reticulocyte is 5% and the red cell indices show hypochromia and microcytosis of mild degree.

Prepared by: ____________ Staff title/Student status ____________

MICHIGAN STATE UNIVERSITY HEALTH CENTER
East Lansing, Michigan 48823

CLINICAL RECORD (PROBLEM-ORIENTED FORMAT)

Date & Time | Patient Name: Miss Mary Blank | Unit Record No. 16711

Assessment: The moderate reticulocytosis probably reflects the effect of iron she has been taking. This may also account for the relatively mild anemia, hypochromia, and microcytosis.

Plan: Further study. We will withhold iron therapy to reduce the chances of intolerance until her diet is stabilized in a day or two, although she has tolerated iron in the past.

John Black, M.D. Medical Intern

MICHIGAN STATE UNIVERSITY HEALTH CENTER
East Lansing, Michigan 48823

CLINICAL RECORD (PROBLEM-ORIENTED FORMAT)

Date & Time	Patient Name: Miss Mary Blank Unit Record No. 16711
1/11/72 4:00 p.m.	PROBLEM #4 Retitled Grief Reaction: Dr. Enelow and Dr. Swisher saw this patient in medical psychiatric conference. It was felt that the specific diagnosis was an adjustment reaction of adult life (grief reaction) and that she had shown great efforts to compensate effectively for her real loss following her mother's death. This was felt to indicate a good prognosis.

It was brought out that she has fears about having cancer "like mother."

Assessment: It is now clear that depression and anxiety are the principal problems from the patient's point of view.

Plan: We are unable to reassure her at present that she does not have cancer, but we have told her that there are several other more likely possibilities to account for her bleeding and that we will know more about this problem soon after she has been seen by Dr. Regis of the Gyn service.

We will give her psychologically supportive care on the medical service, encouraging her to discuss her feelings about her medical problem and life situation. Miss Jones of Social Service will also see her daily, interview her in this context, and assist her with several problems, including renewal of her lease, deciding about sharing her apartment, and obtaining a sick leave. We will not give anti-depressive drug therapy at present.

R. J. Peel, M.D. Medical Resident

6

EMOTIONAL AND BEHAVIORAL RESPONSES TO ILLNESS AND TO THE INTERVIEWER

1 PSYCHOLOGICAL REACTIONS TO ILLNESS

Blum[1] describes ten major reactions, one or more of which is likely to characterize a patient's response to becoming sick. They are: depression and self-rejection; fear; counterphobia; anxiety; frustration and anger; withdrawal or apathy; exaggeration of symptoms; regression; dependency; and self-centeredness. These general emotional reactions are not specific to any particular illness and are separate from the physiologic effects of any particular disease. They are, however, characteristic of that individual's usual response to stress or to anxiety-provoking situations. Later in this chapter we will discuss some ways of dealing with these responses during the interview.

Psychological reactions to illness begin before the indivdual defines himself as sick and before he seeks help. Lederer[2] suggested that the responses of the sick to their illness could be described in three phases: first, the transition period from health to illness; second, the period of "accepted" illness; and third, convalescence. In the transition period from health to illness, Lederer pointed out, most persons first become aware of some undesirable, unpleasant, and painful sensations as well as a reduction in strength and stamina, to which they respond with some degree of apprehension or anxiety. The pattern of response to the initial symptoms is usually the characteristic mode of reaction to anxiety for that person. Some persons will attempt to ignore the threat, "plunge into health," and work harder than ever. Others minimize the importance of the symptoms while still others become irritable or passive and highly compliant. Certain neurotic patients may positively accept illness. Mixtures of some of the reactions often occur.

Once the patient views himself as ill, the usual response is a regressive one, promoted by a combination of the physiological effects of the illness, the social expectations of the sick role, and the psychological needs of the sick person. Lederer characterized the main features of this regression as egocentricity, constriction of interest, emotional dependency, and hypochondriasis.

Whether the patient comes to the doctor's office or medical clinic in the first or second stage of his illness will, of course, be greatly influenced by his culture, socio-economic status, and his usual ways of dealing with anxiety. But at either stage, it is important for the interviewer to recognize these responses, to identify them correctly, and to deal with them or correct for them in evaluating the clinical data.

Anxiety

Every illness produces a mixture of fear and anxiety in the patient. Some of the fears may be realistic such as fear of pain, disability, death, or economic disaster if medical care is prolonged. Usually talking about such concerns to a sympathetic and supportive clinician will help reduce them to a manageable level. The difficulty is that many patients are reticent about their fears. As we discussed in Chapter 2, this reticence tends to vary with the culture or subculture from which the patient comes. Patients who have been taught from earliest childhood to "be a man" or "be a good sport, don't complain" find it very difficult to admit their fears. The necessity for a discreet inquiry about such fears is indicated when the patient does not express it directly but gives indirect evidence of concern.

Since the term "fear" may be unacceptable, it is probably best to ask, "Are you worried about this?" Or, if the patient appears worried, though he has said nothing, it is usually preferable to confront him with a remark like "You look worried." If the patient describes an event or symptom to which fear would be the usual response, but expresses none, a supportive inquiry may be helpful, something like "That must have been frightening."

Anxiety, on the other hand, is usually considered to be a more diffuse feeling of apprehension that is difficult for the patient to attribute to a specific worry or fear. Fear and anxiety co-exist in every illness and are normal or expectable responses.

The most common sources of anxiety are feelings of helplessness; fear of dependency; inability to accept warmth or tenderness; fear of expressing anger.

Helplessness. The paradigm for the anxiety experienced by patients because of feeling helpless is the situation of the surgical patient.[3] No patient feels more helpless. The surgical patient knows that he will be immobilized, possibly unconscious, and during that period in which he can do nothing for himself and nothing to protect himself, a major "attack" will be made on his body. To some extent, every patient feels that there is little or nothing that he can do to help or protect himself. He is in the hands of someone, often not well known to him, upon whom he must depend completely. Further, he cannot really make an objective assessment of the clinician's ability and knowledge. Even the relatively simple procedure of drawing blood or moving the patient from a hospital bed to a cart evokes some measure of anxiety because of helplessness. There are patients who can tolerate helplessness, who have a basic trust in authorities and experts. There are other patients, however, whose self-esteem and feeling of personal worth depends on being active, independent, and aggressive. To be helpless, or to be confined to a bed, creates great anxiety in such persons.

The patient's response to anxiety over helplessness usually is an intensification of his basic style of dealing with anxiety. A typical response is counterphobia. The counterphobic individual reacts to anxiety by denying it and attempting to demonstrate just the opposite by his actions. His response is designed to convince himself and to communicate to others that he is not afraid. The idea that illness could result in being helpless is so intolerable that behavior designed to demonstrate the opposite is acted out.

A forty-two-year-old businessman succeeded in building a large and diversified company largely through his own efforts. He was accustomed to being involved in a number of business deals at any given time and kept constantly in touch with all his operations even having a telephone in his automobile. When admitted to the hospital for examination, though seriously ill and in great discomfort, he was unable to lie in bed. He walked around the room, made business phone calls, and repeatedly interrupted the student who was attempting to conduct an initial diagnostic interview.

The usual indication that a patient is becoming very anxious is an intensification of his customary ways of coping with the world. For instance, the compulsive patient who has a need to be organized and to keep the world orderly and predictable will, on falling ill, become much more compulsive and extremely "fussy." He will insist on even more orderliness, predictability and neatness, or cleanliness than usual.

A twenty-two-year-old college student was admitted to the hospital for examination because of weakness, diarrhea, weight loss, abdominal pain, and evidence of anemia. He was a highly organized, orderly, and neat individual who was described as "compulsive." In the hospital, he complained of failure to collect his stool specimens, and lack of punctuality with schedules, even though neither complaint was warranted. He became upset if he did not receive a new hospital gown each day, even though his was not dirty.

The anxious patient may be difficult to interview until the anxiety itself has been discussed. The patient who fears helplessness reacts best when the clinician's air of competence and concern indicates that he can be trusted; when he feels that he is receiving full and complete explanations in answer to his questions, reducing the ambiguity of the situation; and when efforts are made to reduce his sense of helplessness by allowing him to be as active as the situation permits.

Dependency. The social role of patient means that passivity and reliance on others or, in other words, dependency, is expected. In the reasonably flexible individual, being dependent when one has become a patient does not pose difficulties. It is possible for individuals who are ordinarily quite independent to accept dependence on the physician, nurses, and medical staff when they become patients. But there are individuals whose need to be independent and active is very strong and who have kept up a constant battle to ward off any impulse to be dependent. For them, to be cared for is quite unacceptable. Becoming a patient represents a temptation to them that is very threatening. These are the patients who are most likely to have a counterphobic response to their anxiety. They may put off going to the doctor or clinic, and once there may minimize their symptoms for fear of being ordered to bed.

Inability To Accept Warmth or Tenderness. Blum[1] has pointed out that popular writing in psychology emphasizes the shame which can attend anger and sexual desires but that reluctance to experience tenderness is rarely mentioned. Tenderness refers to sympathetic and affectionate acts by which a person expresses love and concern for another person. Much of the care patients receive from family, friends, and medical personnel is tender care. This makes some people anxious.

Such patients when interviewed, particularly if they are seriously ill and in a hospital bed, become brusque and gruff and speak in distant or irritable tones. Their behavior communicates "keep your distance" and can be upsetting to an interviewer who is trying to be friendly and helpful. It may be necessary for the interviewer to examine his own behavior. To be overly solicitous or warm may be far too threatening to the patient. An increase in the interviewer's own reserve may reduce the discomfort of such a patient.

Fear of Expressing Anger. There are many things that can provoke anger in a patient. A patient who arrives on time for a two o'clock appointment and then has a forty-five-minute wait in the reception room before the interview begins has a legitimate source of anger, for example. Anger can be an appropriate response to many of the circumstances of being a hospital patient. Inattentive personnel and failure to respond to the patient's needs are common, though not always intentional, occurrences in the hospital. But the situation of being helpless and dependent on others makes a patient especially sensitive to failures to meet his needs. Anger is a common response.

However, there are people who cannot permit themselves to express anger. With such a patient, anxiety over helplessness together with a fear of upsetting those on whom he must depend, potentiates his fear of expressing anger and increases his anxiety. This is often reinforced by physicians and nurses whose behavior communicates to the patient that they will not accept his anger and may retaliate. Yet, an important dimension of the clinician's role is to encourage expressions of such anger and to tolerate it even when it seems somewhat unreasonable. Only then can the patient's anxiety over his anger be reduced.

Depression

Schwab *et al.* studied the medical records of patients referred for consultation at the University of Florida Teaching Hospital and found that the term "depressed" could be found in 32 per cent of all the records they studied.[4] It is probable, however, that depression accompanies every severe illness. Research on responses of children to separation from their mothers, on bereavement, and on psychosomatic illness[5, 6, 7] all lend strong support to the view that depression is a psychophysiologic response to loss, including loss of self-esteem. Thus, while depression may be the underlying problem in a large proportion of those patients who consult their physician with complaints of fatigue, weakness, lack of energy, insomnia, backache, or headache; depression as a response to illness is equally common, if not more so. Characteristically, depressed people have feelings of worthlessness, hopelessness, apathy, and guilt together with a profoundly empty or lonely feeling. The depression will be manifested in the patient's manner, tone of voice, posture, and speech. Thinking is slow, speech is sparse, and voice volume is low. Hopelessness and sadness are reflected in the patient's drooping shoulders, downturned mouth, and lack-lustre eyes. A severely depressed patient will volunteer little and will respond to questions with brief, relatively uninformative answers. This will reduce the amount of information that can be obtained about the onset and development of the illness. Many of these patients are people for whom having an illness is equivalent to being useless or "bad." Self-accusation may also be a component in depressive response to illness in instances where a patient believes he has not taken proper care of himself or has ignored advice given to him previously by his physician. Mild to moderate depression can be dealt with relatively easily during the interview, and good interviewing technique may bring some relief of the depressive symptoms. Severe depression can, however, be a major complication of the illness as well as of the interview itself.

Depressive reactions to illness may be characterized by apathetic withdrawal with silences. In such an instance a confrontation can be very helpful. A statement like "You look very sad" or "You look depressed" gives the patient the opportunity to talk about his depressed feelings. It is usually necessary to be more active in interviewing a depressed patient than one would be with other types of patients. More direct questions have to be asked and these are usually asked earlier in the interview than with a patient who is more communicative.

A special problem may be posed by the patient who begins to cry during an interview. Many clinicians find this uncomfortable. However, it may be of considerable help both to the patient and to the interviewer. Fighting tears often results in the patient not being able to speak. Weeping, on the other hand, often affords relief of severe depressive feelings and may make it possible for the patient to resume his account. It may also help the patient to feel closer to the clinician. The appropriate response of the interviewer is to maintain a sympathetic silence while the patient cries and respond with a supportive remark thereafter, i.e. "You must be feeling very bad." A common error, usually stemming from the interviewer's discomfort, is to interrupt the crying with reassuring or supportive remarks before the patient has had a chance to "cry it out." It is better to wait patiently, to provide a tissue if necessary, to respond with sympathetic support after the patient has stopped crying and to make no effort to resume the interview until then.

When a patient is on the verge of tears and this is clearly making it difficult for him to speak, it is often helpful to invite the crying with a confrontation: "You look like you are about to cry." The opportunity to cry followed by the support offered by the clinician will permit the interview to continue and it can be therapeutic.

Denial

There are some patients whose customary way of dealing with frightening ideas or impulses is by never permitting them to enter their minds. On becoming ill, such patients must deny to themselves that such a thing has happened or that they need treatment. Consequently, they minimize or completely deny symptoms, and consciously or unconsciously mislead the interviewer. Such patients are never completely aware of the degree to which they withhold, modify, or alter significant information. Other patients, not ordinarily deniers, will consciously withhold or distort information because they are ashamed or fearful of the consequences of revealing it. Morgan and Engel[8] point out that denial or withholding is usually betrayed by the obvious disparity between the patient's condition and how he reports it. He may overstate how well he feels or be overly vehement about the non-existence of a symptom. A tendency to dismiss all symptoms with such prefixes as "only" or "a little" should cue the interviewer to the fact that the patient is using denial. Those patients who consciously withhold information often respond with evidences of discomfort or embarrassment which reveal that a sensitive topic is under discussion about which the patient would rather not say too much.

Patients who always deal with unacceptable thoughts and feelings by denying them are not reliable informants about their own illnesses. If the interviewer clarifies his role at the outset and can create confidence in himself he may be able to reduce the amount of denial used by the patient. But as Morgan and Engel point out, with this type of patient it is essential to interview a reliable informant as well. They warn, however, that in almost all instances the patient should not be confronted with the information obtained from the outside source.[8]

In subsequent interviews, with the development of a good clinician-patient relationship, the degree of denial used by the patient may be reduced markedly, or in the case of the conscious withholder, disappear completely.

Projection

There are individuals who deal with all perceived internal dangers through projection. They control fear by shifting it from mysterious and potentially dangerous internal events to more concrete, more understandable, and potentially more controllable targets outside themselves, which they misperceive as the source of the danger. Like denial, projection is usually a character trait, though it may be relatively undetectable until the individual begins to become aware that he is feeling ill. Such patients respond to the discomfort and limitation of function that are part of the transition from health to illness by becoming suspicious of everyone around them, including the physician and other health professionals they encounter in seeking help. These patients tend to be distrustful as a matter of course but can tolerate their distrust during communication under ordinary circumstances. However, the internal danger to continued existence that they perceive in illness exacerbates their distrust since much more than usual is now at stake. Interviewing such patients is a difficult task at best. During the interview, the patient may angrily burst out with "Why do you want to know that?" The most insignificant action may be construed by the patient to mean that the interviewer is not to be trusted and can create anger or accusations of bad faith or ill will. The interviewer or anyone who is trying to be helpful may be bewildered and annoyed by such attacks. When a patient becomes clearly suspicious and angry at the introduction of a topic into the interview, the interviewer would be well advised to back off for the moment. The best attitude toward paranoid patients is tactful firmness, avoidance of angry responses to the patient, consistency, and patience. Only in time and with consistency will it be possible to build a sense of trust in the patient, if at all. If all the desired information cannot be obtained in one interview, the clinician must be patient and use as many interviews as necessary to collect the needed data. With the paranoid patient, it is a good idea not to interview collateral sources except with the permission of the patient and in his presence.

2 RESPONSES TO THE DOCTOR

The doctor-patient relationship tends to bring out attitudes and behavior reflecting previous relationships with other authorities or skilled technicians whose competence had an important bearing on the individual's comfort or welfare. This is also true of the nurse and the social worker but probably to a somewhat lesser degree. The more the patient feels that he is sick, and to that extent more helpless and dependent, the more likely it is that his attitude toward the doctor will reflect a great deal of these previously learned attitudes. These attitudes are often manifested in ways that appear totally irrational to the interviewer. A patient who has had an angry, competitive relationship with his father, perceiving the physician as a powerful authority, may become antagonistic, sarcastic, and competitive even though the doctor has done nothing that would ordinarily elicit such a response. Female clinicians often encounter irrational responses based on the patient's early experiences with being mothered.

There is also the likelihood of an irrational response to the doctor, nurse, or other clinician as succorer or sympathy giver. Because the patient is usually in pain, is anxious, and is aware of a threat, possibly of death or at least of impaired function, his need for attention and sympathy is far greater than it is at other times. He is therefore very likely to respond in ways that reflect his relationship with his mother or other individuals to whom he turned for love and sympathy for his childhood discomforts. If these were satisfying experiences, he may be a relaxed and appropriately compliant patient. If they were frustrating experiences, he may approach the clinician with a mixture of fear, suspicion, and expectation of disappointment. If, as is so often the case with individuals who had chronic illness in childhood, the patient obtained attention and sympathy mostly through illness, he may embrace the role of patient and exploit it for as much sympathetic attention as he can get.

Still another determinant of the patient's response to the clinician is the experiences he has had in the past in getting health care. For some people, particularly those raised in urban ghettos who obtained health care in clinics at large public hospitals, the matter of going to the doctor evokes memories of long waits, impersonal and dehumanizing encounters, and disregard for privacy. Chronic illness in childhood requiring painful procedures may make every visit to the doctor a dreaded event.

In other words, the interaction between doctor and patient, as well as between nurse and patient or other health professionals to whom the patient turns for help when sick, is highly charged with emotion. This will significantly affect the patient's interview behavior. Some of the more common responses that can pose problems for the interviewer include silence, over-talkativeness, seductiveness, anger, aggressively demanding behavior, suspicion and distrust, and passive or dependent behavior.

The Silent Patient

With most patients, occasional silences are not uncommon during an interview. Silences of up to half a minute (which may feel quite protracted, even interminable, to the interviewer) usually mean that the patient is trying to recall something, or is silently debating to himself whether to speak about a given topic or not. This is discussed at length in Chapter 3. Many interviewers, and most beginners, do not tolerate such silences well and some interviewers never permit a patient the luxury of a period of silence. This may reflect, in part, the clinician's lack of comfort with the doctor-patient relationship since in conversations with people with whom one has a reasonably close social relationship, silences are not uncommon. It may also partly reflect the clinician's feeling that he has a task to perform, to be carried out with maximum efficiency and dispatch. The most common reason clinicians interrupt silences is their own tension. Most interviewers tend to over-estimate the duration of a silence. A useful exercise is to experiment with estimating the length of timed silences during interviews before actually checking the time. With practice one can learn to permit silence until the patient's tension suggests a confrontation or until the patient speaks.

The patient has been talking about her low back pain. The backache began during her first pregnancy, became worse after her second pregnancy, and is now constant. There is a note of marked discontent in her voice. After a few minutes she falls silent.

(*After about 20 seconds*)

INTERVIEWER: Anything else?

(*Silence—20 seconds. The patient looks more depressed.*)

INTERVIEWER: You look quite unhappy.

(*Silence—15 seconds.*)

PATIENT: I feel just awful. The children are just too much for me. All that lifting and carrying hurts my back so much. And I get no help from Jack. (*Tears appear*) Oh, I just knew if I talked about it, I'd start to cry.

There are patients, however, who remain silent for long periods of time, or fall silent frequently. The interviewer may have the feeling that he is constantly pushing the patient to keep communication going and obtain some information. This usually means that the patient is seriously depressed, which may be part of the illness or a response to it. Questioning about symptoms of depression, as well as careful observation for the classic signs of depression in the patient's facial expression, posture, and attitude, will clarify the diagnosis. Prolonged and repeated silences may also be a manifestation of an organic brain disease or a psychosis.

There are instances when prolonged or repeated silences result from poor interviewing technique. Clumsy or insensitive handling of the opening phase of the interview, too many specific questions asked too early in the interview, too many interruptions, or tactless remarks may result in silences and brief answers which reflect withdrawal and, usually, an offended patient.[8]

The Over-talkative Patient

A most difficult problem for beginner and experienced interviewer alike is the over-talkative patient. This patient may be seen as a barrier to getting a day's work done with reasonable efficiency. He very often frustrates the clinician's efforts to get sufficient relevant information within reasonable time limits, and he is usually a major source of irritation to him. Such a patient, then, slows down the clinician and imposes a burden of self-restraint upon him. This is not, however, the only reason that such patients are irritating to the interviewer. There is usually an aggressive quality to such a patient's communication which has a controlling or dominating effect. One type of over-talkative patient is the obsessional individual who insists on giving an over-detailed account, omitting nothing, not even the most trivial detail. In interviewing such a patient, one must be careful to avoid over-facilitating through encouraging nods, gestures, and phrases. Relatively specific questions should be introduced earlier in the sequence of the interview than might be done with a less obsessive patient. The interviewer should limit his show of interest when the patient is supplying a great deal of trivial detail but show greater interest where appropriate. Courteous interruptions when enough information has been obtained about a given point followed by another question will also keep the interview focused and make it possible to accomplish the interviewing task within a reasonable period of time.

There are patients, however, who will not be hurried. Their obsessive need to recall detail and to present all of it to the interviewer is so great that attempts to focus the interview fail to hasten the patient's account to any measurable degree. Impatience or anger on the part of the interviewer will only complicate the relationship and make matters worse. In such cases, it is best to relax, to accept the situation as gracefully as possible.

> The patient was a forty-year-old obsessive man who was describing the pressure of each job he had after leaving a somewhat subordinate position in a large industry for a series of executive positions with small federally funded community projects. Midway through each such description it became apparent that the pressures were similar and the patient's symptoms were identical each time they recurred. In describing the third recurrence, the interviewer decided to interrupt.
>
> PATIENT: And then the stomach pains began again. First I began to notice that I'd get nauseated after breakfast—
>
> INTERVIEWER: (*Interrupting*) Were the symptoms the same as the first two times?
>
> PATIENT: Oh, yes. (*Goes on to recount them all, once again.*)
>
> The interviewer took a deep breath, settled back, and, glancing at his watch, began to rearrange mentally the remainder of his day.

Another type of over-talkativeness is encountered in the patient who rambles. Often elderly, or simply garrulous, this patient does not behave as an obsessive patient does, but seems to be poorly organized. With this type of patient, one should interrupt when the patient wanders away from the topic at hand unless the patient is in fact supplying information that appears indirectly relevant. Refocusing the patient's attention may be frequently necessary. There is still another type of very talkative patient whose chattering quality betrays his underlying anxiety. A friendly, reassuring, or supportive comment about the patient's evident anxiety is often sufficient to reduce it.

Since for many people verbal communication is a way of controlling and reducing the freedom of the other individual, there is a danger with some patients that the interview can become a battle of the wills. To get the job done, and to reassure the patient that the interviewer is, in fact, capable of carrying out diagnosis and treatment, the interviewer should not allow control of the interview to slip into the patient's hands. On the other hand, an interview should be conducted sensitively enough that the patient does not feel dominated or over-controlled. Most patients respect a clinician whose manner suggests strength and self-assurance. But there are individuals who cannot stand the feeling of being subservient. This, in itself, need not pose a problem. But when such a patient cannot accept a relationship of mutual participation, the relationship can be a severe trial of patience for the clinician.

Not all over-talkativeness represents an attempt to dominate the other person. Some patients feel a kind of closeness when talking. They tend to be lonely individuals who cannot tolerate silence and feel that there is a bond between them and the other if someone is speaking. This is detectable by the interviewer who will feel it as a "sticky," clinging kind of communication. Bed-ridden patients suffering from chronic disease will often make every effort to prolong interviews and keep on talking, fearing that the interviewer will go away.

The Seductive Patient

The patient has certain expectations of the clinician-patient relationship which play an important role in his interview behavior. He expects to have the source of his disorder found and corrected. He expects some degree of comforting or care, some reassurance, and a successful outcome. Sometimes the patient's expectations about the outcome are unrealistic, and no patient likes to hear that it may not be possible to help him.

Some patients may have unrealistic expectations of another variety. They may look for more than a professional relationship. Some may develop fantasies of an intimate personal relationship or even a love affair. And some may behave seductively with the clinician in an effort to make their fantasies come true. Usually such patients are hysterics, or they may be in a hypomanic or manic episode of an affective psychosis.

With the hysterical patient, or with the patient who has become attracted to the physician but who is not psychotic, such seductive behavior will rarely emerge in an open and undisguised way. But there are clinicians who, consciously or unconsciously, foster such unrealistic expectations about an intimate non-professional relationship.

A special problem is posed for every clinician when he finds a patient of the opposite sex very attractive. Young physicians, in particular, may have to cope with their own feelings in response to such patients, though this problem is by no means confined to young people. Older clinicians whose personal or family lives are unsatisfying or in disarray may respond to an attractive young patient with sexual feelings and a desire to convert the professional relationship to a social one. It is important to recognize these feelings, to accept them as a natural response, and to keep clearly in mind that they cannot be acted upon.

In some instances physicians may be seductive by encouraging unrealistic expectations about prognosis. In a misguided attempt to create trust and confidence, one can become overly supportive or misleadingly reassuring. Overdone warmth can be seductive and stimulate fantasies of love or sexual relationships. The clinician should avoid such indirectly seductive behavior as telling his troubles to the patient and seeking emotional support from the patient. It is not wise to use pleasing the physician or nurse as a motivation for cooperating with treatment, as this may stimulate fantasies of personal reward for good behavior. Physical expressions of affection can be very seductive. And, of course, from time to time a clinician and patient do seduce each other, often with disastrous results for the personal lives and families of both.

When a patient is openly seductive or makes direct sexual advances the correct response is a firm, professional one. Without scolding or moralizing, the patient must be reminded of the limits of a professional relationship. If these steps are not taken, explosive complications may result.

The Angry Patient

Another trial of patience for the interviewer is posed by the angry patient. Anger can be a response to illness. There are people who ordinarily can tolerate delay in having their needs cared for but who become short-tempered and irritable when they are ill. They become angry, demanding, and highly critical of the physician or other health professional. One can read between the lines, in the patient's behavior, a communication of fear. The patient is saying, "I am afraid that there is something seriously wrong with me. Are you doing everything you can to help me?" When one feels unfairly attacked, it is a human response to react with anger. However, this will damage the relationship and greatly reduce the possibility of helping the patient. When the patient is angry, one should try to step back and examine what is happening. Warmth, appropriate reassurance, and an open recognition of the relationship of anger to fear is most likely to be helpful.

In other instances, the interviewer finds himself the target of an irrational angry outburst seemingly unconnected with him. Anger may be displaced from an unavailable target (spouse or employer, for example) or from a situation which has just occurred in which the patient did not have the opportunity to express his angry response. For example, a receptionist may have handled the patient in a cold and abrupt manner and turned away without allowing him a chance to voice his anger. In the hospital, a patient may have been treated insensitively moments before by a technician, nurse, or orderly. A little time will permit the anger to subside. A comment like "I find it puzzling that you are angry with me" may uncover the true source of the anger.

Students sometimes become upset when they encounter an apparently irrational angry response from a patient they are about to interview. Sometimes the anger is ascribed by the patient to the fact that it is a student who is about to interview or examine him. This calls for an examination of the patient's anger with him. Here, a confrontation is the best way of proceeding. "You sound very angry" makes the patient's response the opening topic. Some patients, or their relatives, may insist that they are not willing to be interviewed by a student. At such a point, it is best to bow out gracefully and call for help from a staff member supervisor or resident physician.

Of course there are also times when the clinician has provoked the anger himself. Brusqueness, sarcasm, moralistic comments, or attitudes of superiority easily provoke anger. This may be a matter of thoughtlessness or haste. Too often, doctors interview hurriedly because of time pressure. One should always examine one's own behavior before ascribing anger to some difficulty or personality trait of the patient.

Anger can be a defense against the threat of feeling closeness or warmth toward the interviewer. This response may be provoked by the interviewer's overly warm or seductive attitude though it may be aroused in some patients by simple expressions of professional concern. If this is perceived as threatening by the patient, he may react with anger. The threat of feeling warmth or closeness provokes some people to anger in an effort to drive the other person away. Such patients can tolerate receiving help from relatively cool and reserved individuals.

There are individuals whose life style is characterized by anger. They are angry at everyone around them. Even in repose, their manner and facial expression communicate this. The chronically angry man or woman is always a difficult problem for the interviewer. Often his difficulties are related to his anger. The clinician must keep in mind that he is not the primary or sole target of this anger. Observation and the history of the patient should make clear that this is part of the patient's life style and that it is possibly related to the discomfort that brings the patient to seek help.

Aggressive behavior in general is often a means of dealing with a feeling of helplessness or a fear of surrendering to tendencies to be passive and dependent. Some people customarily handle their fear of becoming dependent by maintaining an aggressively independent stance and struggling to maintain control of every situation. For such patients, to become ill increases their fear of passivity and helplessness. They are likely to react with anger to being a patient. When a topic is introduced that touches on an area in which they feel inadequate or where they fear they have failed they are likely to become angry and abruptly dismiss it. It is best not to push for information at this point. If the patient begins to feel that he can safely depend on the physician without completely surrendering his autonomy, he is likely to be willing to supply the information later.

The Paranoid Patient

Occasionally the clinician will encounter a patient who has a paranoid personality. Such individuals are chronically angry, suspicious, and distrustful and they easily become convinced that some person or agency has a malign plan or design directed against them. They tend to brood, become depressed over real and fancied injustices, carry grudges, ruminate about wrongs which were experienced years before, and quickly assume that the clinician's intentions cannot be trusted. Such patients may or may not be delusional but in either case they are most difficult to interview. Any topic which arouses their suspicion, or provokes angry accusations, should not be pursued. Warm and reassuring behavior tends to be threatening to these patients and provokes more paranoia. It is best to maintain a friendly but cool and detached neutrality with paranoid patients. Tactful firmness, avoidance of angry responses to the patient, and consistency help to build whatever sense of trust the patient may be capable of feeling. Reassurance and support, on the other hand, which might be warmly received by most patients, is usually very upsetting to the paranoid patient.

A Note on Evasive, Indirect, and Embarrassed Patients

Sensitivity to the patient's experience in the interview dictates that one may not always proceed at once to the task of gathering data about the patient's present complaints and problems. When a patient shows evidence of evasiveness or indirectness, it is a natural tendency to push harder for information, to make one's questions more specific and more pointed, or to press for more precise and detailed descriptions. This is a mistake. There is, usually, some topic or concern that the patient must get out of the way first. Evasiveness or indirectness frequently means that the patient is ambivalent about talking about something, knowing that it would probably be helpful but fearing to speak openly. The patient may be embarrassed, feel guilty, or fear that something about to be revealed will not be kept in confidence. The skilled interviewer will, at this point, abandon the direct inquiry and shift to a discussion of the patient's behavior and apparent discomfort to reticence. A comment like "You seem to be having a great deal of difficulty talking about this" will often open a discussion of the source of the difficulty. After the discussion it should be possible to continue the inquiry with less reticence on the patient's part. Other patients have difficulty talking to anyone and will require somewhat more direct questioning and specific inquiries to elicit details than the usual patient.

The patient who states early in the interview that he'll be happy to answer the doctor's questions may appear to the inexperienced interviewer to be especially cooperative when actually he is frequently hoping to avoid certain areas of information. His is not a cooperative attitude. He is saying, in effect, "I won't volunteer a thing." Similarly, other patients, basically passive or dependent individuals, have great difficulty volunteering anything and prefer to be led, to be asked questions to which they will supply answers rather than to volunteer information. This is often experienced by the interviewer as demandingness, which is exactly what it is. If the clinical relationship continues, these patients are likely to become more and more openly demanding. It is important for the clinician to understand the reason for the demand and to maintain an appropriate distance. In this way he will be able to avoid becoming angry and possibly punitive.

Social Distance

The interviewing task is considerably more difficult when there is a great deal of social distance between clinician and patient. The problem lies on both sides. The patient's reservations, ability to trust, and ability to cooperate will be influenced by the attitudes he brings from his culture and his social class to the physician-patient relationship. The patient of low socio-economic status sees the upper-middle-class professional much as he sees all persons of a higher status rather than purely as a helping person. Similarly, the clinician, no matter how hard he may try to transcend this distance, will carry attitudes into the interview that reflect his feelings about the patient as a representative of his class or cultural reference group. The physician, nurse, social worker, or other health professional who interviews a patient must examine himself carefully for the ways in which his attitudes, prejudices, and values are preventing him from being first and foremost the patient's advocate and helper. He must also learn to correct for those attitudes, suspicions, and behavior that reflect the patient's social and cultural origins.

3 EMOTIONAL ASPECTS OF THE PHYSICAL EXAMINATION

If a well-conducted interview has preceded the physical examination, a relationship has been established. The physician is no longer a stranger but a concerned individual who is trying to be of help. The physical examination is one more step in the data collection process. Without such an interview, the physical examination is an invasion of the patient's privacy and may even be experienced as a humiliating assault.

Disrobing in front of someone else is usually done in intimate situations with a trusted person. Naked is almost a synonym for defenseless. For this reason, the fully clothed physician must always be aware of the problem of shame, embarrassment, and feelings of inferiority that his unclothed patient may experience. He should permit the patient his dignity by seeing to it that he is properly draped. He should be polite, business-like, and not linger over especially emotion-laden areas like breasts, genitals, and rectum; but he should not be so swift as to suggest that *he* is embarrassed. Alertness to evidence of shame, embarrassment, and guilt feelings is most important. If such feelings appear to be upsetting the patient or interfere with the conduct of the physical examination, a discreet inquiry or confrontation can lead to a discussion of the patient's feelings and a reduction in their intensity.

For some patients, the physical examination provides an opportunity to be seductive. Appropriate professional reserve and the presence of a nurse or attendant usually suffice to forestall any overt attempts to make the doctor-patient relationship a sexual one, but the physician should be aware that his own behavior can stimulate erotic fantasies in certain patients.

The patient may also have anxieties about specific areas of the body. If these are not detected in the interview, they can easily be seen during the examination in the patient's remarks as a given area is approached. This gives the examiner the opportunity to gather more data and the patient a chance to bring his anxieties out into the open. A simple confrontation: "You sound like you're worried about your (heart, bowels, or other area approached)" will usually suffice to bring out the patient's concerns or fears. The principle is this: interview and examination are not clearly differentiated separate processes. The interview is still in process during the physical examination.

REFERENCES

1. Blum, R. H., *The Management of the Doctor-Patient Relationship.* New York: McGraw-Hill, 1960.
2. Lederer, H. D., "How the Sick View Their World," *Journal of Social Issues,* 8:4-15 (1952). Reprinted in E. G. Jaco, *Patients, Physicians and Illness.* Glencoe, Ill.: The Free Press, 1958, pp. 247-256.
3. Enelow, A. J., and M. Wexler, *Psychiatry in the Practice of Medicine.* New York: Oxford University Press, 1966, pp. 267-271.
4. Schwab, J. J., F. R. Freemon, R. S. Clemmons, and M. L. Scott, "Differential Characteristics of Medical Inpatients Referred for Psychiatric Consultation: A Controlled Study," *Psychosomatic Medicine,* 27:112-118, 1965.
5. Spitz, R., "Hospitalism, An Inquiry into the Genesis of Psychiatric Conditions in Early Childhood," *The Psychoanalytic Study of the Child,* 1:255-278, 1945.
6. Bowlby, J., "The Nature of the Child's Tie to the Mother," *International Journal of Psychoanalysis,* 39:1-23, 1958.
7. Engel, G. L., *Psychological Development in Health and Disease.* Philadelphia: W. B. Saunders, 1962.
8. Morgan, W. L., and G. L. Engel, *The Clinical Approach to the Patient.* Philadelphia: W. B. Saunders, 1969.

7

INTERVIEWING CHILDREN

Ray E. Helfer, M.D., William B. Weil, Jr., M.D., and Mary Ryan, M.D.

1 INTRODUCTION

Though the basic goals of the pediatric interview are identical to those of the interview with an adult patient, that is, gathering data and establishing a helping relationship, there are some significant differences. One rarely works with the patient alone; most commonly it is with the parents also, and sometimes with siblings. Gathering data secondhand increases the likelihood of distortion and the difficulty of evaluation.

Consequently, a number of questions arise, such as what do you do with a child while you are speaking to his parents; from which parent do you gather data; should both parents be present during the interviewing process; are the child's answers to questions reliable; when do you perform the physical examination; what do you do with a crying child; do all the parties concerned, including the doctor, agree upon the actual problem?

The short attention span of children, the large number of interruptions, and the questions and concerns of parents create still other differences between interviews with adults and those with children.

2 SOURCES OF INFORMATION

The Mother

The mother of the child is usually the person who can provide the most data about the child's problem. She has, however, particular personal needs that must be recognized and dealt with during the interviewing process. Most often, she not only wishes to please the physician and tell him what he would like to hear but also tries to present herself as a "good" mother. This need often interferes with her ability to be objective in providing the necessary history. She may repress certain unpleasant events. If the family is large, she may also have difficulty sorting out facts regarding one or another child. She often has a significant problem in recognizing certain physical handicaps and mental defects in her child. The interviewer may become impatient with a mother who is unable to provide him with accurate, objective data if he fails to recognize these pressures on her to present herself as a "good" mother and her child as a "typical," "average," "good" youngster.

The Child

Inexperienced interviewers, and those whose experience has been mainly with adults, often fail to take children seriously as sources of information about their own ailments. A student observed by one of us in another setting spent thirty-five minutes gathering a history of abdominal pain in a twelve-year-old girl from a mother who spoke very poor English. He failed to realize that the child, who spoke perfect English, could give him a much more detailed history of her complaint than could the mother. Throughout the whole interview, he did not ask the child a single question.

Although many children find it difficult to talk with older people, significant data can be obtained by observing them interact with their parents and at play. One can sometimes use the play room to advantage in obtaining accurate data by asking the child,

"Where does your dolly hurt?" or "Where does your dog hurt?" relating the question to a toy the child is holding. As children grow older they become very accurate in their reports of personal discomfort. They often provide this information with a candidness that is unusual in the adult. Directing one's attention completely toward the parent or the child usually impairs communication.

Optimally, the interviewer should see the parents and the child alone, as well as together. On occasion the parents may feel inhibited in the presence of the child and vice-versa. The child usually has a strong need to please the parent. It is almost impossible, for example, for a child to relate a history of being mistreated because of his underlying need to please those who care for him. Even if the child is interviewed alone, he may not be willing to tell the interviewer everything that is happening to him at home.

The Father

Fathers rarely have detailed knowledge about the day-to-day health of their children. But the father does play an important role in determining whether or not the advice of the physician will be carried out. He should not be overlooked during the interview. If the situation requires only a brief interview and the mother can provide all necessary information, the father should be brought into the instruction or follow-up phase of the interview so that he can participate in carrying out the recommendations.

If the child's health problem is complex, it is sometimes helpful to collect specific data from both father and mother. This is best done in separate interviews so that the observations of each can be compared for completeness and accuracy. Conducting separate interviews as well as a combined interview, though time-consuming, may make it possible to assess the closeness of the parents, their individual interpretations of the information given to them, and whether or not they expect to carry out the recommendations. This may be worth doing if the clinician suspects serious problems between the parents that are part of the child's health problem. Joint interviews often bring out unsuspected specific problems. The interviewer may learn that the child's original complaint was merely a guise under which one or both of the parents could seek personal help. Interviewing the families of children who are ill is discussed in Chapter 8.

3 BEGINNING THE INTERVIEW

The setting in which the interview takes place is even more important with children than adults. Attention must be given to the child's needs and desires while the clinician and parents are talking. Children who are old enough can be given something to do, such as drawing, coloring, and building with blocks. Supervised play areas can be provided. Interviewer and parents can then talk in a more relaxed atmosphere. But the setting should not require the parent and child to be separated during the entire session. Significant information will be obtained by observing the parent and child interaction during the interview and physical examination. A child will be much more cooperative if he has been active and stimulated rather than ignored during the interview process.

The opening moments of an interview, if handled properly, can set the stage for a close working relationship between doctor and family. Observations of medical students interviewing mothers in a busy pediatric clinic have indicated specific problems of beginners with the first few moments of the interview. Many students fail to introduce themselves. Very few students ask the mother how *she* is getting along. A very common error is to fail to pay any attention whatsoever to the child. Obviously, the manner in which the interviewer introduces himself, explains his role, and expresses an interest in both the parent and the child during the first few moments of the interview is highly correlated with the character of the relationship established. This, in turn, has an important effect on the amount of data obtained.

The interviewer should permit the parent to determine the exact point at which she wishes to begin the discussion. An open-ended question such as "How is everything going?", "Are you having any problems with your child?", "Tell me why you came today?" is helpful. As the interview proceeds, it should follow the same principle described in Chapter 3—that is, the interviewer's specific information-seeking activities should be those that exercise the least control first and the highest degree of control as late in the interview as possible. Specific information should be sought through direct questioning only after the parent has been given ample opportunity to express her concerns and questions. Beginning the interview with "Tell me your chief complaint" is unwise as it usually narrows the focus of the interview too early, possibly excluding significant data.

The interviewer must remain extremely flexible and not become concerned if circumstances necessitate that he change his usual procedure. It is often necessary, for example, to interrupt the interview and begin the physical examination early. An astute clinician will observe that the child is becoming extremely restless and that any further delay in the physical examination may result in a hyperactive and uncooperative patient. The child may become tired and irritable if the examination is delayed too long. The many interruptions that occur while collecting data from parents and children require that the interviewer take care not to overlook some of the needed information. It is unusual to be able to collect all relevant data during a single session. Physicians who are accustomed to highly structured interviews are frequently uncomfortable in this situation.

Parents who bring their children to a health care setting usually have in mind specific questions which will usually come up during the course of the interview. Specific answers should be provided, if possible, at the time the questions are asked, even though they appear to interrupt the interviewing process. This strengthens the relationship with the parent. The pediatric interview like all interviews is a reciprocal process. Not only does the doctor gain information but also the patient and parents obtain support and reassurance, and the parents get specific answers to many questions they have about the child's health.

4 OBTAINING SPECIFIC INFORMATION THROUGH DIRECT INQUIRY

The Family History

The history of the immediate family should begin with data about the parents' health. A general inquiry should be made first, using an open-ended question referring to family health first. The current health status and major health history of the grandparents and all siblings should be obtained in all instances. Any unusual health history in other members of the family should also be noted and may indicate the need for establishing a detailed family pedigree.

If the family is new to the interviewer or clinic, the mother's history should be obtained in considerable detail beginning with her own growth and development, the onset of her menarche, her first marriage, her first pregnancy, and each pregnancy thereafter. The information on pregnancies will vary somewhat with the specific problem at hand but in general should include a brief chronological statement about the mother's health during the pregnancy, its duration, the date of delivery or other termination, the birth weight of the infant, immediate postpartum problems, and information about the postnatal course of the baby. Inquiry into contraceptive practices is useful as this will often provide information as to the planned or accidental nature of the pregnancies. An appropriate medical history of household contacts should also be obtained.

Family Histories in Genetic and Growth Disorders

In collecting diagnostic information about a child, the family history is often of special significance because of the frequency with which genetic disorders are first encountered in children. Also, the early determinants, or precursors, of many adult diseases can be ascertained during childhood. If there is any reason to suspect a significant familial or genetic disease pattern, it is helpful to develop a full family. pedigree. This should include, as a minimum, the ages, present health status, causes of significant morbidity or mortality, for the siblings, parents, parental brothers and sisters and their offspring, grandparents, and great grandparents. If any significant pattern of illness or of a genetic trait is noted in developing the pedigree to this extent, one should then explore the same information for the siblings of the grandparents, their offspring, as well as siblings of the great grandparents and their offspring. It is often not only time-saving but also valuable for clear recording and analysis to make a diagram of the pedigree with the informants at the time the history is taken. In this way, one can attach correct names to each individual in the pedigree and be sure of the exact relationships of the people involved. This is of great assistance when additional family history is obtained at subsequent interviews.

Additional history should be obtained in the care of patients with growth disorders or nutritional disturbances. The stature and body habitus as well as socio-economic class and ethnic origin should be determined for as many family members as can be identified. A history in comparable detail is useful in many other disorders such as diabetes mellitus, malignancy, allergy, in which there may be genetic factors.

Past Medical History

The pregnancy from which the child patient was born is of great significance. One should inquire about the mother's prenatal care, its source, frequency, and the stage of pregnancy when it was begun, as well as the character of the labor and delivery. Not only will significant medical information be obtained, but this line of inquiry can be fruitful in eliciting parental attitudes toward sexuality, health-care–seeking behavior, and family life in general. Frequently parental attitudes toward individual children have their origin in the circumstances around the pregnancy from which a particular child was born. Such information is often useful in understanding complex behavioral patterns later in life.

The newborn and infancy period of the patient should then be evaluated in chronological order. It is helpful to obtain information on the birth weight and neonatal course of the patient. The specific details of this are frequently not available for children in large families or for older patients. The duration of hospitalization at the time of birth both for the infant and for the mother may be an indicator of the presence of neonatal problems and may prompt an examination of the hospital records.

At this point, the history can be further developed chronologically from the neonatal period up to the patient's present age or a series of specific inquiries can be made about nutrition, illnesses, accidents, hospitalizations, immunizations, personal habits, and general development. The choice of one of these two approaches, or of a combination of the two, is usually made at the time of the interview and is based on the interviewer's sense of what problems seem most pressing. In either case, information should be obtained in each of the above noted areas in most situations. In infancy, it is important to know if breast feeding was attempted, for how long, and with what success. The types of feeding formulas that were used, how frequently they were changed, and for what reason also should be determined. The immunization history is most easily obtained while discussing infancy. Information about later booster immunizations should not be forgotten.

Illnesses, poisonings, accidents, and injuries are subjects of importance in the pre-school child. Since this is the period when weaning, toilet training, mealtime behavior, and bedtime behavior are established, information on each of these experiences should be sought. These areas may prove to be highly sensitive. Tact and sensitivity are called for in obtaining this history. The facts about these behaviors are important, but even more important are the parental concerns and attitudes toward their establishment.

Entering school begins another period of transition for the child. His age and the circumstances under which he began school should be determined. The school child's learning experience, school progress, and the changing character of his relationships with siblings, parents, peers, and adults may be points of significance. The problems presented by adolescent patients are discussed later in this chapter.

The Developmental History

Proper evaluation of a child's development requires a sound background of information about normal human growth. Not only physical growth, but growth of cognitive function and development of motor skills and of social emotional behavior are important. Information in these areas can be obtained both from open-ended questions and from quite specific ones. One might begin by asking a parent "Tell me about your daughter's growth and development." If this does not elicit the information sought, one might become more specific and ask, "What did she weigh at birth and at one year of age?" Knowing about a period of growth failure may lead to the discovery of important events that took place in this child's life which might not otherwise come to light. On the other hand, if a child at age twelve is normal in physical size and psychosocial development, and is entering the early stages of adolescence, little may be gained by a detailed evaluation of physical growth from birth up until age twelve. A more general question, "How has Bill grown?", would quickly establish whether a growth problem existed in the past. Similarly, a child of normal growth who is having no difficulty with his school work in a grade appropriate for his age is unlikely to require a detailed investigation of his early cognitive development or feeding habits.

Although aspects of physical growth other than height and weight may be of importance in evaluating a child, most parents are unlikely to remember these features unless a complex or unusual problem occurred. Exact height is rarely recalled. Often the only method of establishing a history of linear growth is to ask parents to compare a child with his siblings, with other children of comparable age. The accurate history of birth weight and weight gain is much more likely to be available. This is the period that most families will consider when asked about physical growth. To save time, when there is no major concern about growth failure, the information being obtained can be checked against commonly accepted normative values to determine the need to go into more detail. Average birth weight is approximately 7½ pounds. By one year of age, weight will ordinarily have tripled; by two years, it will have quadrupled; and by four years the average child weighs approximately 40 pounds and is 40 inches tall. If necessary, height measurements can usually be obtained from the records of other physicians, public health programs, schools, and camps.

The major phenomena of motor development, sitting without support, crawling, standing, walking unaided, running, and climbing stairs are events that most parents recall. The age of walking unaided is probably the most frequently remembered since it is often a cause of anxiety. Language development is also well recalled by most parents. Excessive weight gain is much less likely to cause anxiety on the part of the parents than is failure to gain weight, although it may ultimately be worse for the child.

In adolescence growth reports may be a cause of concern. This is particularly true of growth and development of sexual characteristics of adolescence. The girl with an early but normal growth spurt may be of more concern to parents than the girl with delayed growth. In boys, late physical growth is commonly of more concern. The development of sexual characteristics when early or late in either sex generally provokes anxiety. Knowledge of normal variations will assist the interviewer in understanding parents' reactions.

System Review

The general principles developed in Chapter 4 apply in the pediatric interview. However, there are several differences between the system review in a young child and in an adult. First, the complaints, particularly those which are subjective, are frequently interpretations by the parents. For example, hematuria may mean red urine as seen either by the child or the mother. It may also be reported to the mother by the child, with the mother then interpreting the child's report as hematuria. In general, open-ended initial questions in each area of the system review are likely to obtain valuable data.

Complaints are poorly localized and vague in the small child. Small children may be less able to localize sensation, even though the pathological process itself may be reasonably well localized. For example, almost all children localize any abdominal pain to the periumbilical area. Urinary tract infections in a small child are more commonly manifested by fever, malaise, and anorexia than by dysuria, incontinence, hesitancy, and urgency. When directing questions to the child it is important to communicate at his level. Using phrases such as "Does your belly ache?", "Do you hurt anywhere?", "Does it sting when you pee?", may prove helpful.

6 SPECIAL PROBLEMS ENCOUNTERED IN PEDIATRIC INTERVIEWS

On occasion it will be necessary to interview a mother who has taken several children for care to an office or a clinic. Should separate interviews be conducted with each child? This will be answered by considering the available time and the nature of the problems presented. When a child is very ill or in great discomfort, he is usually taken in alone. When several children are taken, some of the data can be collected simultaneously about all of the children. A convenient method is to place each child's name at the top of a column on a sheet of paper and record specific information that is given by the mother under the appropriate name. Many questions regarding illnesses and past history can be handled by this method. Specific concerns which the mother has about one of the children will have to be dealt with individually. It is usually not feasible to carry out separate detailed interviews with each child a mother takes for care on a given day. However, the physician and mother must constantly keep in mind the individuality of each child, give him individual attention and talk to him when his turn comes to be examined.

When a health worker is involved in interviewing the mother of a seriously ill child, early and specific judgments must be made regarding the urgency of the situation to determine the appropriateness of gathering unrelated data at that time. It is frequently appropriate to deal with an acute illness by immediately gathering the information pertaining to the problem and complete the interview at a later date. The student should not feel uncomfortable if he finds it necessary to break up his history-taking process to deal with a particularly acute problem.

Gathering data from a parent who speaks poor English may create significant problems. One often finds that the child himself can give appropriate and accurate data. In some situations, where the child may not be a good historian, he may be able to serve as the interpreter.

The pediatric hospital ward would seem to be an ideal setting in which to obtain a child's medical history. The child can be cared for in bed and the parents and doctor can remove themselves to a quiet room for the history-taking. Although this has several practical advantages, a major disadvantage is that the physician fails to observe the interaction that takes place between the child and his parents. For this reason, part of the history should always be obtained while the parents and child are together in the same room. The pediatric ward does provide an opportunity for the history to be expanded and broadened as parents visit during the period of hospitalization.

The ambulatory care facility, on the other hand, does not lend itself to this continuous history-taking process. Little time is available to gather a rather large amount of data. In this setting, it is quite feasible to use auxiliary health workers to gather information in specific areas. These workers can save significant time for the physician by determining developmental status, gathering past medical history and records, immunization records, and similar data while the parents are waiting to see the physician.

A specialty clinic operating within an ambulatory care facility presents particular problems that must be clearly recognized. The tendency here is to collect only very special data regarding a specific problem. Continued general health surveillance must be assured for patients who attend only specialty clinics.

Physicians frequently are superficial in interviewing parents and children they know well and when dealing with a problem they know well. When asked to care for a neighbor's adolescent daughter with a sore throat and earache, a physician may give a superficial interview and examination and fail to recognize a major problem, such as an unannounced pregnancy.

Parents commonly introduce subtle cues throughout the interview referring to emotion-laden or embarrassing problems which they would like to have the physician bring up or discuss. These include such things as bed wetting, masturbation, sexual activities of adolescents, and school problems. The interviewer must recognize these cues and follow up with appropriate leading or specific questions. Beginning interviewers often tend to avoid this cueing by the mother. One student, for example, aware that he should ask about the child's behavior in school, asked, "How is your child doing in school?" The mother responded by saying, "Well, he is having a little problem." The student's next question was, "Tell me more about his cough." That particular student, as do many of his colleagues, felt uncomfortable about gathering data concerning the child's behavior and avoided the need to deal with this problem, once it was disclosed.

6 THE ADOLESCENT PATIENT

As the child approaches adolescence, his relationship with the clinician changes even as it is changing with the other members of his family. In early adolescence, the young patient may come to the office or clinic with a parent and this is often accepted because transportation is needed. The emerging young adult may even resent this necessity. His need is to be seen as an individual becoming independent of his parents.

The adolescent must know with certainty that the physician from whom he seeks help is acting on his behalf and not in the interest of his parents. On the other hand, it is not possible, or wise, to disregard the parent in most situations. Whatever is told to the parent must first be discussed with the patient, thus assuring the maintenance of the physician-patient relationship. Parent contacts may be vital in preserving strained family relationships, though the clinician should always remember that the patient's needs are his primary consideration. At times a three-way interview between parent, patient, and physician may open lines of communication between a parent and patient and allow a full discussion of the problem. This is not advised in the initial interview, prior to the establishment of a good relationship between clinician and patient.

Basic interview skills differ little from those used with adults. The principles in Chapter 3 can be followed with good effect. There are some differences, however.

For one, to a greater extent than most adult patients, the young patient will often need to get to know the physician before he divulges his grave concerns. At times, several office visits will be made with minor or even fictitious illness, which tends to alienate the busy private practitioner. The patient may sense this and begin to search elsewhere for care. For this reason, patience and a willingness to take time with the young patient are necessary. If the physician understands this, he may offer several things: frequent unstructured office visits, including a complete physical; truthful explanations of the problems the patient recounts, neither minimizing his symptoms nor offering a placebo; the avoidance of moralizing; and a willingness to look for clues to the patient's real concern when posed a question about a "friend" or an off-hand inquiry about some "minor" concern. Occasionally the clues are obvious: "By the way, doctor, what do you think about talking in your sleep? I've heard that some people that have seizures do it." Or, "While I'm here, would you mind looking at this silly spot on my skin?" Once the clues are identified, concerns can be dealt with quite directly. The adolescent will come more quickly to the point with a confrontation like "You act like you are worried about cancer," rather than "Are you worried about cancer?" Opening up these worries for examination and discussion brings relief to the young patient. Often more problems will be spilled out at that time. Even if they are not, a relationship has been established which leaves open lines of communication for the future.

Another difference is that adolescents do not tolerate silence as well as older adults. When a young patient falls silent, the interviewer should make some facilitating, supportive remark. In general, one should be more supportive with younger patients. The supportiveness must, of course, stem from a genuine liking and concern for the patient. Adolescents are usually quick to spot a "phony" attitude. But support and reassurance should not be used in such a way as to limit the patient's emotional expressions. Overly sympathetic and premature expressions of support and reassurance tend to inhibit the patient's communications about his feelings. When a patient is talking freely and with feeling about his worries and concerns, silence is always best until he has expressed himself fully.

Some, though by no means all, adolescents are suspicious of older people. Those who have specific difficulties with older authorities will approach the clinician with a defensive hostility. The wise clinician accepts this behavior and permits the expression of suspicions or anger. He does not return the hostility, nor does he withdraw. Instead, it is well to make them the subject of the interview by confronting the patient with his behavior in a calm accepting way. In this way, trust can be built and the underlying fears and confusions permitted expression.

8

INTERVIEWING THE FAMILY

Cyril M. Worby, M.D.

Most clinicians consider the individual patient to be the object of their primary concern. Occasionally, the patient's family comes to the foreground, sometimes at the clinician's request as a source of specific information, sometimes as a result of the family's request for information and reassurance. These encounters between clinician and family often tend to be unplanned, episodic, and focused on an immediately pressing issue. Not infrequently, the encounter is awkward for all concerned.

Yet on many occasions the clinician's concern should go beyond the individual patient to include the family as a whole. In this chapter, the circumstances in which interviewing the family can be useful will be discussed and some techniques described.

1 ENCOUNTERS AROUND NON-CRISIS EVENTS

Much of the clinician's interaction with patients and families occurs at times of crisis, but this is by no means always the case. A seemingly routine matter may provide an opportunity to influence the future health of a person and his family through a family interview. Such opportunities occur at a number of points in the life cycle of the family.[1] Even before the family is formed, for instance, there is the premarital examination. Because most states require a medical statement concerning absence of venereal disease, premarital examinations by a physician are common. According to Nash and Louden, "Many leading physicians . . . indicated that the premarital examination provides an opportunity to extend preventive medicine to the new family unit. Therefore, they suggest that its scope be increased to include a general physical examination, including a pelvic examination when desired, and sexual and contraceptive counsel."[2] By providing an opportunity for the couple to discuss questions and feelings about sexuality, contraception, independence from in-laws, and the division of responsibilities in the home, the physician may help strengthen the relationship.

The prenatal care of the woman in her first pregnancy presents another opportunity. The husband should be invited with his wife for one or more of the prenatal visits. Unfortunately, clinicians rarely regard man and wife as a couple and as a new family in the making. Consequently, an important opportunity for the physician to identify problems and provide support is lost.

After the child is born, the father's presence with the mother at the well-baby checkup, whether conducted by the nurse-clinician or physician, can provide an opportunity to detect early evidence of a strained relationship between parent and the infant and between the parents themselves. Differences between parents often arise over such questions as: Should the infant be allowed to cry? Is it safe to have a baby sitter? Who should pick up the baby in the middle of the night? These differences may stem from a couple's profound anxiety about their capacities as parents and about the fragility of the infant, as well as from feelings of competitiveness with the infant. The alert and sensitive clinician uses such questions as a way of opening a discussion of the parent's anxieties, providing an opportunity for support and reassurance.

There is another opportunity for a family interview when the child is to begin school for the first time, since many school systems require a physical examination and statement of immunization from a clinician. Most often this is a perfunctory affair, carried out as rapidly as possible by the clinician. But the first child's entry into school is a major event in the life of the family. The occasion of this physical examination permits a glimpse into how the family is functioning at this stage.

Ruth, an only child, is six and soon to begin first grade. She is brought by her mother for the routine pre-school exam. The clinician notes that the mother talks to Ruth as one would to a much younger child. During undressing and dressing, he notes that the mother does more than necessary for the child, and a struggle develops around Ruth's wanting to do some of it herself.

After stating that the physical exam is normal, the clinician asks, "How do you and your husband feel about Ruth starting school?" The mother replies, "I don't know what I'll do with all the time on my hands. My husband travels a lot and it gets lonely. I'm afraid it will get worse when Ruth starts school. He's been offered a job with much less traveling and he's thinking about it. I've talked with him about my getting some part-time work, but he's not sure he likes the idea."

The clinician replied that Ruth's starting school would require readjustments likely to affect the welfare of mother, father, and child. He suggested that Ruth's mother and father make an appointment to talk about this. The mother said she thought it might be a good idea but didn't know how her husband would feel about it. After talking it over with her husband and finding that he agreed, she made an appointment. The parents spontaneously brought up their concern that Ruth seemed younger than other children her age. The clinician asked the parents why they thought this might be so, and the mother volunteered that she might have babied her too much. The clinician was able to suggest a number of ways in which the parents could encourage Ruth's increasing autonomy. He also was able to help the parents discuss the issues between them—the husband's job and the wife's increasing leisure time. The husband later decided to take a job requiring less travel and the wife and husband were able to agree that the wife would take a part-time job on a trial basis.

Not all clinicians are interested in this kind of involvement because of time constraints or personal preferences. But it may be unnecessary for the clinician to interview the family himself. It can be done by another member of the health care team. Increasingly, clinicians are working in close association with allied health professionals such as social workers and psychologists. When psychosocial problems such as family difficulties complicate issues of health care, this collaboration can be very valuable.[3]

2 ACUTE HEALTH CRISES

Sudden illness is a common event that creates anxiety in both the patient and his family. Some illnesses are very frightening even though they are unlikely to have serious consequences, such as obstructive laryngitis in a child requiring a tracheostomy. Illnesses with acute onset and high probability of serious disability such as severe burns, heart attacks, and strokes are very stressful to the family. The sudden death of a family member will most likely have a major impact on the family.[4]

> Mr. J., a forty-one-year-old assembly-line worker, married father of a twenty-year-old daughter and fifteen-year-old son, was awakened from sleep with crushing sub-sternal pain radiating down his left arm. He felt nauseated and feared he might die. His wife called an ambulance. He was taken to a local hospital and placed in the intensive care unit. A coronary occlusion was diagnosed. His hospital course was characterized by several life-threatening episodes, during which the outcome was uncertain. Nevertheless, he recovered and was discharged from the hospital in thirty days. While in the hospital, he reflected on his harrowing experience. Will this happen again? When might it happen? Will I survive the next time? Is there anything I did wrong which led to this? Is there anything I can do to prevent this from happening again?
>
> Upon her husband's return home, Mrs. J. was constantly afraid that he would over-exert himself and suffer another coronary. She became overly solicitous, hovered over him, found it difficult to leave him home alone, and drastically altered the meals served in

the home, feeling that if everyone followed her husband's diet, he wouldn't be tempted to stray from it. Their sexual relationship was affected for fear that "something might happen." After her husband returned to work, Mrs. J. still felt insecure about the future. In both obvious and subtle ways, she was having difficulty tolerating the increasing independence of her children. For example, she opposed her daughter's engagement on the grounds that "this isn't a good time for it."

The episode of acute illness in this example was resolved, leading to complete functional recovery from the cardiovascular standpoint. The intrafamilial consequences, however, were not resolved. They persisted beyond Mr. J.'s recovery from the heart attack, altering the family's relationships with one another in profound ways. A series of family interviews during and after hospitalization would have provided an opportunity to express anxiety and to receive support, realistic reassurance, and education about diet, exercise, and other matters related to Mr. J.'s rehabilitation.

3 SLOWLY EVOLVING HEALTH CRISES

Other health crises may develop slowly but remain at a crisis level for a long time. Chronic, progressive renal failure and irreversible cardiac decompensation, for example, are health care situations in which family interactions and decision making become a major concern to the clinician.[5, 6, 7]

Jane F., aged eighteen, married in her third month of pregnancy. She had been living at home and in her senior year in high school. Her husband, Arthur, aged nineteen, had graduated the year before and was working in a gas station. Their relationship dated back two years. Arthur was particularly sympathetic to Jane's increasing desire to become independent of her parents, who tended to regard her as a little child, incapable of making her own decisions. Following marriage, they found a small apartment. They quarreled a good deal over Jane's inconsistent behavior toward her parents: at times she asked them to mind their own business; at other times she seemed to invite their involvement in minor matters.

> Jane gave birth to a normal appearing girl without undue complications. Jane's parents seemed to regard the newborn baby as their own, coming over without invitation, offering advice on how to care for the infant. This led to increasing friction between Jane and Arthur. Toward the beginning of the second month after birth it became clear that something was seriously wrong with the baby. She was not developing properly and her head was getting large. Studies revealed that the infant had hydranencephaly. There was absence of cerebral hemispheres, blindness, spastic extremities, and obstructive hydrocephalus. The prognosis offered was several months of life at most, and it was recommended that the infant be institutionalized. Jane's parents at first refused to believe the diagnosis and prognosis, then accused Arthur of being responsible, claiming that he didn't treat Jane well during the pregnancy. Jane felt torn between her parents and Arthur and couldn't make a decision about what to do with the baby, whether to institutionalize her, care for her at home until she died, or give the baby to her parents for care.

In this case a newly established nuclear family was experiencing great conflict with the extended family when a health crisis occurred. Through family interviews, which in this situation would include Jane, Arthur, and Jane's parents, some clarification of issues and feelings might have been attempted.

In chronic renal failure, treated by hemodialysis or kidney transplant, the involvement of the family is essential. Dietary and fluid restrictions for the dialysis patient and the medical regimen imposed on the transplant patient require the understanding and cooperation of all family members. Changes in the family role of the patient, who can no longer carry on as wife-mother or husband-father as in the past, create problems for all. Family interviews can be most helpful in developing the necessary alterations in family functioning.

4 DIAGNOSTIC PROBLEMS

Data-gathering and diagnosis may be aided through the family interview, particularly when patients are unable to communicate (for example, patients with dementia, delirium, or in coma). At times, severe pain or profound depression interferes with a patient's capacity to communicate. The family may be able to give crucial information in such circumstances.

> A five-year-old girl was noted over a two-week period to undergo behavioral changes characterized by irritability, insomnia, and confusion about her surroundings. She also developed a staggering gait. A brain tumor was suspected and the child was hospitalized for diagnostic evaluation. In the course of evaluation, high levels of lead were discovered in the blood and urine. In an interview with the parents no obvious source of lead, such as peeling paint, could be pinpointed. During a subsequent interview, the clinician mentioned a number of possible sources of lead poisoning, one of which was insufficiently fired glazes in ceramic vessels. The parents recalled that the girl was given a brightly colored ceramic cup as a present several months previously. The cup became her favorite and she consumed all of her liquids from it. Analysis of the cup revealed a high yield of lead. This was the source of her poisoning.

This is a simple example of information about a family member that had to be obtained from other family members. In some circumstances the whole family, including the patient, works with the clinician to bring out data or piece together a story clarifying the diagnostic problem.

> Mr. A., a fifty-two-year-old postal worker was admitted to the hospital with fever of 101°F., cough, breathlessness, and frontal headache. He gave a one-week history of fatigue, anorexia, backache, and increasing cough. Physical examination, x-ray, and laboratory studies pointed to a diagnosis of viral pneumonia. Over a period of three days his condition worsened in the hospital.
>
> The clinician, encountering the family members at the bedside, decided to review their recent activities with them. The patient had reported having no pets in the house. The family members, in reconstructing their activities in the recent past, recalled that a few weeks earlier Mr. A. had spent a day with a friend who was a pigeon fancier. It was winter time and the birds were in the basement. The

two men spent the day repairing cages. This information enabled the clinician to make a presumptive diagnosis of ornithosis. After drawing a blood sample for acute serum tests, antibiotic therapy was initiated with good results within several days.

5 MANAGEMENT PROBLEMS

There are times when the diagnosis is clear, the treatment objectives unambiguous, and the procedures straightforward; yet, repeatedly, and unexpectedly, things go wrong. The clinician's attitude may shift from perplexity to annoyance. This state of affairs may arise in such chronic illnesses as diabetes, ulcerative colitis, intractable epileptic disorders, and asthma.[8, 9] In such situations, the problems usually are an outcome of processes that involve patient, family, and clinician in complex interactions which often are best clarified through bringing the whole family together for discussions.

> Jack, a sixteen-year-old only child, had been followed by his family physician for a grand mal seizure disorder over a three-year period. The seizures were well controlled with dilantin for the first two years. During the past year, for reasons unclear to the clinician, seizures would occur in an apparently random fashion, despite trials of several combinations of anti-convulsants. The boy finally "confessed" to the clinician that he sometimes fooled his mother, who gave him his medication, by pretending to swallow the drugs. He didn't quite know why he was doing it; he did say, "she is always hassling me" about being careful and not doing the kinds of things other boys his age were allowed to do.

This is an example of a family conflict complicating the patient's treatment. The next step would be for the clinician to meet with parents and son to discuss their relationship. Many patients whose treatment requires daily medication will express anger toward other family members by failing to take medication and thus precipitating symptoms. Some children can induce their seizures by looking at the sun and waving their fingers before their eyes. They can sometimes be helped with family therapy.[10]

6 THE SCOPE AND CONDUCT OF THE FAMILY INTERVIEW

When a family interview is contemplated, the clinician should have a clear idea of what his goals are. Is his purpose to gather data to help make a diagnosis? In that case his approach is guided by his concern for eliciting information about the patient. If his purpose is to give information, he should present the facts as honestly and realistically as he can and then give the family an opportunity to react and to voice their questions and concerns. If his purpose is to get data about family interactions and processes, he will limit his information-seeking activities to the most open-ended ones and give every family member the opportunity to become relatively spontaneous with each other and to talk about common concerns.

In the care of many patients the interviewer's goal may vary with the phase of illness.

> While driving, a woman skidded on an icy freeway, sustaining serious injuries to her head, abdomen, and extremities. She was admitted to the hospital in coma and in shock. She underwent emergency surgery because of bleeding from a lacerated spleen. As a consequence of her head injury she remained comatose in the intensive care unit. She finally regained consciousness and was transferred to the orthopedic ward for continued treatment of her leg and arm fractures. She remained in traction for several weeks and was discharged home considerably improved, with arrangements for rehabilitation on an outpatient basis.
>
> The nature of the clinician's interaction with this patient's family varied with the phase of the hospitalization and treatment. Eight hours after admission, the attending surgeon who had removed the bleeding spleen met with the patient's husband and mother in the waiting room adjoining the intensive care unit. The nurse assigned to the patient was with the surgeon. He introduced the nurse and explained the nature of her role in the patient's care. First the surgeon gave the husband and mother information, that is, an assessment of how things stood, what had been done, and what was going to be done. He did not minimize the situation, nor did he burden them with the spectrum of possible problems he was required to con-

sider. He prepared them for the inclusion of other clinicians such as the orthopedic consultant. He then invited them to voice any concerns they might have. The husband and mother asked a number of realistic questions, to which both the surgeon and nurse responded. The surgeon noted the tremulous quality to the husband's voice and made the supportive comment, "This must be a very trying time for you." The husband began to weep. So did the patient's mother. The nurse and surgeon nodded in sympathy but did not attempt to interfere with the expressions of emotion. The husband and mother soon regained control. The surgeon and nurse prepared to leave, each indicating to the family how and when they would stay in communication with them.

Three days later, after the patient had regained consciousness, the nurse saw the husband, the mother, and the patient's two children in the waiting room. By now, the nurse had had repeated contacts with the husband and mother and was an important source of information and reassurance for them. But this was the first time the children had been brought to the waiting room. The nurse talked with them and found that they were worried about their mother's progress. It became clear that the father, in his own distress, had assumed the children knew more than they did, and together the nurse, father, and patient's mother helped them to understand the situation.

This example might be characterized by a few brief statements: several clinicians met with the family; the interviews took place in the waiting room of the hospital; the patient was not involved in the interviews; and the clinician-family contact was infrequent and brief.

In other situations, the clinician-patient and clinician-family relationship extends over a long period of time.

A thirty-eight-year-old television repairman consulted his physician. "I can't make my right hand go where I want it to go and I've dropped my soldering iron a couple of times. It scares the hell out of me." Examination revealed incoordination of the small muscles of the right hand. The patient was seen by a neurologist ten days later, but by then complete function of the hand had returned.

Physical examination and laboratory studies were entirely normal. The neurologist called the referring physician, reported his negative findings, and concluded on the basis of the history that multiple sclerosis might be suspected but could not be proved.

The clinician was faced with a dilemma. What should he tell the patient, who was now feeling quite well? If the episode was a symptom of multiple sclerosis, they were dealing with a disease process notorious for its variability in clinical course and severity. The patient might not experience any further symptoms for ten years. On the other hand, he might suffer a serious relapse within several months. Furthermore, there was no specific treatment for it. Consequently, the physician decided to tell the patient that he was uncertain about the cause of the transient symptom. He advised the patient to return for checkups at six-month intervals. After two such checkups the patient had reported no difficulties, so the frequency of the return visits was changed to once yearly.

Four years after the initial episode, the patient called to report weakness in his left leg starting three days previously, and double vision which had begun that morning. Neurological studies over the next several weeks led to a diagnosis of multiple sclerosis. Although the patient's vision had returned to normal, his left leg became progressively paralyzed. The patient remained at home, unable to work. During a phone conversation with him, the physician learned that the patient's wife was very upset over his illness and was asking all sorts of questions which the husband couldn't answer. The physician said that he would come to the home on the afternoon of the next day. He also suggested that all of the family members be there, "so that we might all talk together about the meaning of your illness." The patient responded, "You mean the kids, too?" "How old are they?" the physician asked. "Thirteen, eleven, and nine," replied the patient. "Yes, they probably have been quite worried about you, wondering what's going on and afraid to ask." The patient agreed that this made sense.

After arriving at the patient's home, the physician sat down with the family in the living room. "What do all of you think is wrong with Dad?" asked the physician. After a minute of silence, the eleven-year-old boy said, "He's had a stroke, like grandpa had last year." "No, that's not so," the mother said. "Any other ideas?"

asked the physician. "Does he have cancer?" asked the thirteen-year-old boy.

It soon became apparent that each person in the family had a different idea of what was wrong. For one thing, the issues were so charged with anxiety that communication between the parents and children and between the parents themselves was vague, incomplete, and often cryptic. Family members, including the patient, operated on the assumption, "the less said the better." For another thing, whatever information was openly shared tended to be interpreted by each individual in his or her own private way. The individual's private interpretation was influenced by his or her fears, age, and past experience.

The physician said, "I want to explain to all of you what is wrong with Dad." He was not only speaking to the children, but to the parents also. "First, he does not have cancer or a stroke. He does have an illness which affects some of the nerves which control some of his muscles. Sometimes the nerves heal themselves, which is what happened four years ago, in which case the muscles work as well as before. Sometimes the nerves don't get better, in which case the person has trouble using that part of the body which is controlled by the affected nerves. No one knows what causes this illness. In Dad's case, it doesn't look as if his leg will get better. We hope it won't get worse and we will try to help him adjust to his handicap. Often a person with this illness doesn't have any more trouble for many years, which we hope will be the case with Dad."

Through this approach, the physician served as a model for discussing anxiety-laden issues directly and openly. He also presented information about the illness to all of the family members simultaneously so that they would share the same information. Distortions of this information by any individual within the family might then possibly be corrected by another member of the family. When faced with a health crisis, families may welcome the opportunity to discuss and try to deal with the crisis as a group. The family unit itself may have most of the resources required for coping with the health crisis.

A common disease that may require the clinician's interaction with the whole family for a protracted period of time is metastatic cancer.

Mrs. Coles was forty-eight years old at the time of the family interview. She had had her breast removed two years previously because of cancer. The cancer recurred in her liver and she developed a deep depression of psychotic proportions.

She was treated first with antitumor drugs on the Medical Service, discharged home, then readmitted to the Psychiatric Service for her profound depression. The following interview took place on the day before her discharge from the Psychiatric Service. Her psychiatrist, social worker, the patient, her husband, and her twenty-year-old married daughter were present. Her twenty-three-year-old married son was unable to come.

Following the initial greetings, the clinician began:

DOCTOR: Well, how have things been for all of you?

DAUGHTER: All right. I have my cold. (*laugh*)

PATIENT: I have a nice family. We are very close, in spite of the fact that my son couldn't come up. We are very close because we're very small.

HUSBAND: He works shift work and it is rather difficult for him to get off. And due to the fact that they just had a baby, why they have been more or less tied up in their own little problems and consequently Tom hasn't been to see mother very much, since she's been here. That's the reason.

PATIENT: He hasn't been up at all, to tell the truth.

DAUGHTER: Well, I've only been up once, but mostly because there was only an hour, you know. And I thought he'd like to come up and I came up once. So—that was all.

PATIENT: But I have no brothers and sisters—no aunts, uncles, cousins. I have nobody but immediate family, so we are very close. I mean—well, that's all I have. Just my children and my husband—that's the only family I have. My parents are both dead. I never had any brothers or sisters. Well, I have some relatives that live not too close. Never see them. Once in how many years?

HUSBAND: Four or five years, perhaps.

Note how little was said by the clinician, beyond the open-ended question, "Well, how have things been for all of you?" The question was deliberately put to the whole family at the outset. This is a way of establishing an important ground rule in the family interview, namely, that everyone has the right (and at times, the obligation) to participate in the discussion.

As the interview proceeded, the family continued to justify the son's preoccupation with his own family's affairs since their first child was overdue and there had been two miscarriages previously.

SOCIAL WORKER: Everything happened at once?

PATIENT: Yeah, so they had their own problems at that time. So it was kind of rough.

HUSBAND: And they felt, and I also felt, that—ah—with problems on both sides, it would be quite a clash if Tom and Alice were to try to see Mother, too, having those problems at that time. As you say, everything just happened all at once.

DOCTOR: How do you see that as a clash?

HUSBAND: Well, their problems with the pregnancy and the trouble as Mary just said. And Mother having her problems, all at one time. Just wouldn't fit, that's all.

DOCTOR: Too overwhelming?

HUSBAND: Oh yes.

PATIENT: Especially at that stage of pregnancy. The water broke, you know. That's pretty nerve-wracking, just to be waiting after that.

HUSBAND: What I really mean is that one should not burden the other. The way I felt, the two problems just didn't mix—they would affect mother and, on the other hand, mother would be affected by what was happening there.

PATIENT: I think I was unaware of what was going on.

HUSBAND: Well, yes, you were, you were. But I'm speaking in terms of . . . supposing you had been told about this. You see, this could have had a very ill effect on my wife.

PATIENT: Sometimes I think Dr. Smith thinks I don't like my grandchildren or something. But that is very much untrue.

DOCTOR: She was just saying she does not have much family, but it's growing.

PATIENT: I'm crazy about my first grandchild, he's eighteen months —her son. But I'm just wild about him, and I'm looking forward now to getting acquainted with my other one, my new one.

It is worth pointing out the nature of the clinician's interviewing behavior: "Everything happened at once?", "How do you see that as a clash?", and "Too overwhelming?" These facilitations were aimed at clarifying and encouraging the speaker to expand on feelings and perceptions which were not only relevant to the family's present situation but might be predictive of the family's behavior in the very difficult future. In the next excerpt, the clinician asks the patient directly about the onset of her illness.

DOCTOR: When were the first signs you weren't feeling so well?

HUSBAND: I've been asked this question before and I have found it rather hard to go back in my memory to the exact time.

DAUGHTER: It *is* hard. It was more or less—so gradual.

DOCTOR: Maybe Mrs. Coles could remember.

PATIENT: I had my breast taken off, you know.

DOCTOR: That was when?

PATIENT: A couple years ago. And I lost my father with cancer of the esophagus. When he was forty-seven, he died. Well—I was forty-seven. (*laughs*)

DOCTOR: When?

PATIENT: I'm forty-eight now. I just turned forty-eight and I had that awful feeling that I was going to die when I was forty-seven because he had and I had cancer. After all, this was malignant and they had performed the radical operation and all, the whole thing, the whole muscle and everything. And I had a morbid fear that they hadn't gotten it all and I was going to die and I think that's what started it. And it kept building up, of course, after the operation. While I'd been informed and told by both doctors, the surgeon, and my family, doctor assured that they had got it all, that there was nothing to worry about. And they *finally* had convinced me before I went to the hospital this time that there was nothing to worry about. Well, then they start all these other tests and then, when they found out I had it in my liver; well, then that was it. After all, I had just got to the stage where I was beginning to believe I was going to live for a while, you know, and then to have them tell me I had it in the liver. And they didn't pull any bones, they told me I had it. I mean, they took a biopsy. I was conscious, of course, while they took the biopsy. They just froze, you know. Took a biopsy. And I knew what they were looking for and they told me what they had found. They didn't pull, you know—

DOCTOR: Did you, Mr. Coles, and you, Mary, know what your mother was feeling, was thinking about all this time? Did she let you in on it? Did she share her thoughts with you?

HUSBAND: Well, of course, I knew all this before she was told about it, you see. And naturally I suppressed all emotion when I was with my wife, I didn't let on that I knew any of these things, you know. It made it rather difficult for me. Well, after leaving the hospital, my emotions just broke, as my daughter will tell you. Of course, I knew it. And they told me they were going to tell her.

The direct question that begins the above passage is addressed to the patient, but the husband and daughter start to answer for her. It is not uncommon for one family member to speak for another in a family interview. The interviewer should always note this, particularly when it is repetitive and seems an attribute of family functioning. By saying, "Maybe Mrs. Coles could remember," the clinician encouraged the patient to speak for herself, hoping to discourage the rest of the family from regarding her as "the helpless one."

As the interview proceeds, the patient graphically describes her identification with her father's illness, her fear of a recurrence following initial surgery and her despair over discovery of liver metastases. The clinician asks the husband and daughter if they knew of the patient's turmoil in order to learn how open they may have been to signals of distress communicated by the mother. In such circumstances a conspiracy of silence often develops. The family members may wish to avoid upsetting each other, but they can make the seriously ill person feel increasingly isolated.[11] In the family interview the clinician may attempt to reopen communication to whatever degree the patient and her family can tolerate it.

PATIENT: Well, as I say, I just got over feeling I was going to die with the breast, and then to have—. Of course, when they took the liver scan, you know, that's when they apparently found some signs of it. And, well, it was pretty frightening, you know, to think that you had something like this someplace. I didn't know where it was or how it was. I heard that you don't operate on a liver. You don't remove a liver like you can a breast or something, and you're just stuck, more or less with it, you know. Of course at the time I didn't know they could treat it the way they are treating it.

DOCTOR: So it was hard for the two of you, Mr. and Mrs. Coles, and I assume for you, Mary, also, to talk about this? It was such a—.

DAUGHTER: That I'll agree. I'll tell you something right now. This is the first time she has said anything in front of me, although I knew. But she never mentioned it when she was home. Never, never said anything about it at all. This is the first time she has said anything in front of me at all about it. The first time she has said anything—

PATIENT: I came home from the hospital and I wasn't myself.

DAUGHTER: No. Well, I stayed with her. In fact, I think I handled her more than he did. So, she seemed to be pretty good with me.

PATIENT: I was terribly depressed when I went home from the hospital and I didn't want to go home.

HUSBAND: No, she fought going home.

PATIENT: Oh, I didn't want to go home, Doctor. Why was that? When they told me I was going home, I just—I didn't think I was ready to go home.

DAUGHTER: That's all she'd say.

HUSBAND: I think it was the fear of leaving the hospital and the care she'd been receiving, knowing she wouldn't be able to get that same care at home. However, the care was not needed, the doctors informed me, and there was *no* reason why she couldn't go home, so I—

PATIENT: I felt like I'd lost my last friend when they sent me home.

SOCIAL WORKER: The hospital being kind of a friend, so to speak?

PATIENT: Uh huh. And having what I have—

HUSBAND: That first night at home was like a nightmare—I sat up all night long with her. So the next morning I called Dr. Smith and explained the situation, and he immediately prescribed an anti-depressant capsule which I picked up.

DAUGHTER: No, that wasn't until afterwards. You had to give her those sleeping pills, the ones that really knocked her out.

HUSBAND: Oh, those sleeping pills, yes.

DOCTOR: You must have been scared.

PATIENT: I was.

DOCTOR: You must have panicked.

HUSBAND: She was. She had some rather bad moments all night long.

PATIENT: I was just petrified. I was frightened, afraid of being alone. And, as I say, I got all that attention in the hospital. I had all that care and then to just be sent home on my own.

DOCTOR: Did you think you were that bad off?

PATIENT: Yes, I thought I was going to die–soon. (*laughs*)

DOCTOR: Soon? What gave you that feeling, Mrs. Coles?

PATIENT: Because they couldn't operate, and they couldn't operate on my father, either. And, of course, in the esophagus. I think they can do something for that now but this was twenty odd, some years ago.

DOCTOR: Twenty years?

PATIENT: Uh hmmm. It was twenty-three years ago, because my son was born the same year he died. And they couldn't operate. They didn't say why, but at that time they couldn't. They discovered it at an early stage, and he just had to go on living, of course. I saw him wasting away. Of course, it being there, he couldn't swallow and he went–he had weighed 170 some pounds and when he died he weighed only 98, and he was just skin and bones–an awful, tragic thing to see somebody you love waste away like that. Well, I had that memory, you see, and that's why I was so petrified. And that's why I was so petrified when I even got it in my breast. Of course, in the breast there is more hope for you because they've done wonderful things and I've heard of people who have lived twenty some years after a breast operation, but then when I found out that I had it internal. Then I was just thrown for a loss. I was just petrified. And then when they said they were going to send me home–(*laughs*)

DOCTOR: You figured they gave up on you.

PATIENT: Yes, I just figured they would send me home to die, see? Now I can talk about it. I couldn't talk about it before. I was so scared, I couldn't even talk about it.

HUSBAND: This is the first I actually heard her talk about it.

DAUGHTER: Uh huh–

SOCIAL WORKER: Is this new to you, too, talking freely like you do?

HUSBAND: Yes.

DOCTOR: You know, this inability to talk with each other must have made all of you feel very alone and separated.

HUSBAND: Well. Of course, I was able to talk with my daughter.

DAUGHTER: We talked back and forth.

HUSBAND: Son, son-in-law, daughter-in-law.

PATIENT: But just that word.

HUSBAND: With others.

PATIENT: I say, just that word.

DOCTOR: Pardon?

PATIENT: I say, just that word "malignancy" is enough to scare me. If I hadn't experienced what I did with my father, it probably wouldn't have been so bad, but it was so tragic to see him. And he had died at home and stayed at home most of the time, because there was nothing they could do for him. So he just said—he wanted—he was in a nursing home for awhile, and he knew he was going to die and he said, "Well, if I'm going to die, I want to be in my own home." So he was months at home wasting away. And he wouldn't go to bed until he was in a coma. He didn't stay in bed. He said, "As long as I'm alive and I can get up and around, I'm going to get up and walk," and he did. And he didn't go to bed until four days before he died. He was in a coma four days.

This excerpt dramatically illustrates how difficult it had been for the family to share their feelings about an event which was terrifying to them. As a result, they tended to avoid one another. When they were together, their relations were strained by the effort to avoid forbidden topics and feelings. A family interview before the patient's discharge from the Medical Service might have helped prevent this bottling up. It might have reduced the terror and abandonment which the patient experienced within hours of her discharge from the hospital. This terror was communicated to the whole family; it undermined their own capacity to cope and in turn compromised their ability to give the patient support.*

* Interview excerpted from work in progress in collaboration with G. R. Babineau, M.D.

7 CONCLUSION

Under some circumstances, and for variable periods of time, the family as a group rather than the family member identified as the patient becomes the object of the clinician's inquiry. This shift in focus from the patient to the family may be perplexing to the family. Thus it is important for the clinician to make clear the goals of such a shift in focus to the family.

In the case of Jack, the sixteen-year-old boy with grand mal seizures, this would be very important. From the parent's perspective, Jack has seizures which are no longer being controlled. They look to the clinician to solve the problem. They are unlikely to be aware that their relationship with Jack is a crucial factor. Jack has a different perspective. He is annoyed at his mother's coddling. He feels that his parents overestimate his fragility and underestimate his competence. The clinician's task in this case is to help bring the unspoken issues to the surface, to provide a neutral and informed opinion concerning what Jack can and cannot do, to see that therapy is administered, and, finally, to suggest workable ways for the family to resolve differences in perspective that may arise in the future.

In the family interview the large number of verbal and nonverbal events that commonly occur may seem overwhelming to the clinician. This apparent chaos, however, can take on meaning and order if the clinician begins to look for recurring patterns as the interview proceeds. These patterns may be relational in nature, that is, who speaks to whom, who supports whom, what alliances are formed between members, which members seem to be fighting.[12] Communication patterns also reveal a great deal about the family.[13] How are things said? Are communications clear and unambiguous or are they convoluted, unclear, full of multiple interpretations so that the listener is perplexed as to what is meant? Patterns of expressing feelings also emerge in the family meeting. Does a family handle affection and anger in a characteristic way?

The building of trust between the clinician and family presents a different challenge than in the individual interview. Most often, the clinician meeting with the family will have a special relationship with one or more family members. Particularly if there is conflict in the family, the clinician will need to conduct himself in an impartial way, avoiding taking sides and trying to bring out everyone's perceptions of the situation.

The conduct of the family interview can be very gratifying if the clinician is aware that despite the sense of fear, hurt, and even despair that may often be found in families experiencing a serious health crisis, most families have deep resources to draw upon in helping one another.

REFERENCES

1. Worby, C. M., "The Family Life Cycle: An Orienting Concept for the Family Practice Specialist," *Journal of Medical Education,* 46:198-203, 1971.
2. Nash, E. M., and L. M. Louden, "The Premarital Medical Examination and the Carolina Population Center," *JAMA,* 210: 2365-2369, 1969.
3. Cokin, M., E. Colligan, and R. Ferrer, "Helping Parents in a Pediatric Clinic," *Child Welfare,* 50:504-509, 1971.
4. Salk, L., "Sudden Infant Death: Impact on Family and Physician." *Clinical Pediatrics,* 10:248-249, 1971.
5. Simmons, R. G., K. Hickey, C. M. Kjellstrand, and R. L. Simmons, "Donors and Non-Donors: The Role of the Family and the Physician in Kidney Transplantation," *Seminars in Psychiatry,* 3: 102-115, 1971.
6. Korsch, B. M., R. N. Fine, C. M. Grushkin, and V. F. Negrete, "Experiences with Children and Their Families During Extended Hemodialysis and Kidney Transplantation," *Pediatric Clinics of North America,* 18:625-637, 1971.
7. Eisendrath, R. M., "The Role of Grief and Fear in the Death of Kidney Transplant Patients," *American Journal of Psychiatry,* 126: 381-387, 1969.

8. Jackson, D. D., and I. Yalom, "Family Research on the Problem of Ulcerative Colitis," *Archives of General Psychiatry,* 15:410-418, 1966.
9. Green, J., "Self-Induced Seizures," *Archives of Neurology,* 15:579-586, 1966.
10. Libo, S. S., C. Palmer, and D. Archibald, "Family Group Therapy for Children with Self-Induced Seizures," *American Journal of Orthopsychiatry,* 4:506-509, 1971.
11. Norton, J., "Treatment of the Dying Patient," *The Psychoanalytic Study of the Child,* 18:541-560, 1963.
12. Wynne, L. C., "The Study of Intrafamilial Alignments and Splits in Exploratory Family Therapy," in N. W. Ackerman, F. L. Beatman, and S. N. Sherman (eds.), *Exploring the Base for Family Therapy.* New York: Family Service Association of America, 1961, pp. 95-115.
13. Singer, M. T., and L. C. Wynne, "Communication Styles in Parents of Normals, Neurotics and Schizophrenics," *Psychiatric Research Reports of the American Psychiatric Association,* 20:25-38, 1966.

9

DISCUSSING FINDINGS AND PLANNING TREATMENT

1 DISCUSSING THE FINDINGS

At the conclusion of a diagnostic interview, the patient expects to be given a summary of the findings. In most instances, he will want to know about the prognosis, whether treatment is to follow and what it will be. There are exceptions, of course. Some patients do not want the responsibility of sharing knowledge of the nature of the problem nor do they wish to have any responsibility in the treatment. They may even try to prevent a discussion of the findings and planning of treatment. Others will want to know as much as possible, often more than the physician knows at that point. In all cases, however, the interview should be terminated in such a way that further studies, if needed, or treatment procedures, if they are to begin now, can be carried out successfully. This means involving the patient responsibly in a collaboration.

The Discussion

The discussion should open with a frank and clear statement of what the physician has found, in sufficient detail to give the patient an understanding of the problem. The significance of the findings should be explained. At this time, too, the physician should describe the areas of uncertainty for which more data is needed and describe what must be done next, such as laboratory tests, other diagnostic procedures, and further observation.

A common error in this phase of the interview is the use of medical parlance in presenting the information. Ordinary, non-technical language should be used and simple analogies employed to clarify physiological processes being discussed. Vocabulary appropriate to the person's socio-economic status and education should be used. A particular problem faces the clinician in explaining findings to a patient who is from a culture with which he is unfamiliar or who uses an idiom that is foreign to the physician (such as the ghetto black, or the chicano) or to one who has a rudimentary grasp of English.

A complete discussion of the findings does not, however, mean overloading the patient with information. Findings of dubious relevance should be omitted. Throughout the explanation, the physician must be alert to the patient's response to ensure that his explanation is being understood.

There are many patients who consider it impolite to interrupt the physician, to ask questions, or to reveal that they did not understand the explanation that was just given. In a study of doctor-patient communication done at Michigan State University, a well-mannered, smiling, middle-class widow in her sixties was given a deliberately over-detailed and confusing explanation by her physician. Throughout the explanation, she nodded in polite agreement, occasionally echoing a word or phrase and said, "Thank you, doctor," at the conclusion. The physician then asked, "Now, do you understand Mrs. R?" "Oh, yes, doctor," she replied sweetly and respectfully. Gently, but insistently, he said, "What did I just tell you?" She blushed and became quite embarrassed. Only with difficulty was she able to admit that she had become lost very early in the explanation.

The lesson in this is that one cannot be sure from the patient's manner alone that he has understood your explanation or your instructions. At the conclusion, it is necessary to inquire.

An inquiry about the patient's feelings and any questions he may have is also necessary, since, first of all, any explanation, discussion, or recommendation relating to illness will evoke some anxiety and perhaps a mixture of emotions in response. Second, unless they are very passive or handle anxiety by denial, patients will almost always have some further questions. The inquiry should begin in an open-ended way, perhaps something like an encouraging gesture inviting the patient to speak. If facilitation fails to elicit a response, the physician can ask directly, "How do you feel about this?" It is important to permit the patient to express his anxiety, worry, or any other emotional response he might have and to encourage him if he has difficulty expressing it.

When a patient does express his feelings, the most appropriate response from the physician is support. This gives the patient the comfort of knowing he has a concerned physician. Of course, if the patient expresses fear that is unrealistic, that is, about which the physician can honestly give reassurance, he should do so.

Some patients who express their feelings of fear and concern when encouraged to do so may hesitate to ask questions. Blum points out that clinic patients, in particular, rarely ask for detailed information about their condition, and that the less general information a patient has, the less he will ask for. He comments,

> "The self-perpetuation of ignorance on the part of the patient who does not ask the doctor any questions is probably related to cultural, social class, and personality factors. It is reasonable to expect that the more the patient views the doctor as a stranger in language, custom, or outlook, then the less likely will the patient be to begin conversation. It is also likely that the more the patient is afraid of the doctor, or the more inferior the patient feels to the doctor, the less likely will the patient be to ask questions. The regrettable consequence is that communication problems will be greatest with people who need the information the most: people from different cultures, the lower class, or unreasonable and uncooperative people."[1]

Having, therefore, described his findings in clear and non-technical terms; indicated areas of uncertainty and of insufficient information, and what further procedures may be needed; clarified, as much as the information at hand permits, the significance of the findings; facilitated expression of the patient's feelings and responded supportively; the physician must find out if the patient understands. Does he remember what the physician has said? Is it clear to him? The physician should never fail, at this point, to ask "Do you have any questions?" If the patient does not understand what his situation really is he will be unable to participate responsibly in his treatment.

The Patient's Response

Patients' responses to the discussion of findings vary considerably. Some responses represent an attempt to shut off communication. The healthiest response is, of course, a desire to know the situation. Blum[2] describes a few characteristic responses that make for management problems if not dealt with effectively. He calls these: "I don't want to know, so don't tell me," "reassure me," and "prove your love." To these, we would add the counterphobic response and overdone "good and reasonable" behavior.

I Don't Want To Know, So Don't Tell Me

This statement may be made directly by the patient, or expressed in his attitude, in which case the patient is not hearing what the doctor says though he may superficially appear attentive. It comes from patients who are fearful of taking responsibility for their future, preferring rather to depend entirely on the physician. This response makes it difficult to carry out treatment successfully. Accompanied by a certain amount of flattery of the doctor, if not overdone it may lull him into overlooking the attitude and failing to deal with it by confronting the patient. The physician now may be maneuvered into the position of protecting his patient from reality and encouraging the patient's dependency. In such cases, after confronting the patient with his behavior, it is often possible to engage him more responsibly in his treatment.

Reassure Me

The plea for reassurance, as Blum points out, is an invitation to make a promise which, though reducing the patient's fear of an unfavorable outcome, may be impossible to keep. While an honest reassurance in the form of a conservatively phrased prediction can allay anxiety, this sort of prediction often cannot be made after the initial diagnostic examination. This may be because more data is needed, or it may be that the outcome is in doubt and could be unfavorable. In any event, support is more important than reassurance at this point even when reassurance is honestly given. The clinician should clearly express his ability to appreciate how the patient must feel, his concern, and his intent that all possible appropriate diagnostic and treatment procedures be brought to bear on the problem. Reassurance tends to cut off further communication from the patient about his fears or worries with a risk of giving the doctor an unwarranted feeling that he has solved the problem of the patient's apprehensiveness.

Prove Your Love

Jokes are made about the physician's instructions to the patient to go to bed, take two aspirins every four hours, and drink plenty of fluids. They reflect the fact that many patients are disappointed if they don't get some medicine or a "shot." The "prove your love" response, often expressed in a disappointed, "Aren't you going to give me some medicine?"—a request for visible proof of the doctor's concern for the patient is most likely to occur when simple supportive measures or no medication is indicated.

There are physicians who regularly give antibiotics for upper respiratory infections, whether or not they are indicated, to "prove their love" and to satisfy the patient. Others use vitamins or minor tranquillizers this way. Still others deliberately prescribe placebos. In our opinion placebos should be used with great discrimination. It is true that some patients reason primitively and cannot grasp that they can be appropriately cared for even though no medication is given. But most patients respond positively to a sensible discussion that shows respect for their intelligence, and there is then no need for pretense in the form of placebos. We don't want to "addict" patients to medical care and to unnecessary medications, nor to suggest that an answer to all discomfort can be found in a pill or a "shot." Many a drug-dependent individual has been trained to be so by a physician who used his prescription pad too freely. The capacity for self-help and knowledge about when it is appropriate to consult the health care professional cannot be cultivated by prescribing placebos. Educating patients about medication and its overuse is an important part of patient care.

Counter-phobic Response

This is a variation on the theme of "I don't want to know, so don't tell me." The patient's fears are similar, but his response is to deny that he is ill or needs help." "Nonsense," he says, "I'm not ill, nor am I helpless. I don't need you at all." His anxiety that illness could result in helplessness is so sharp that he will behave in ways that demonstrate to himself and others that he is far from helpless. These are the patients who ignore the doctor's advice and prefer do-it-yourself medical care. Breaking through this defensive wall is possible when the patient has consulted you on his own initiative. Confronting him with his attitude makes a realistic discussion possible. If he is reluctantly following another's advice, or has involuntarily become your patient because of a medical emergency, it is very difficult to get him to recognize his underlying anxiety. Whenever possible, the clinician should aim to make the patient aware of his attitude through confrontation given supportively and he should help the patient express his anxiety. This can lead to a realistic discussion of the patient's situation.

Overdone "Good and Reasonable" Behavior

Some patients who are frightened of illness take a "good child" stance when threatened by it. They make no demands, express no fear, and behave as though the physician were unusually skilled and unquestionably able to banish illness. They respond, verbally and non-verbally, with, "Anything you say, doctor. I fear nothing because you are my doctor. I will make no demands on you and will follow your orders completely." Such patients are afraid that to burden the physician with their apprehensions and concerns will annoy him. They feel that they can influence him to exert all his magic and rescue them, if he really likes them. As a result, their psychological distress is not relieved because they are afraid to communicate their fears. Fear is usually reduced by the simple measure of expressing it to the other in a helping relationship. When the physician thinks of such a patient as a "good" patient because of this obedient attitude he may fail to help the patient express and face his anxiety.

This is why the physician must be alert to the patient's verbal and non-verbal response and identify it even as it is happening. This is another way of saying that the task of data collection and evaluation is not discontinued during the discussion of findings and planning of treatment. Rather, observation of the verbal and non-verbal cues about the nature of the patient's response should be a primary concern during the discussion. If the patient is distressed, and responds in one or more of the ways described above, the physician should discuss his feelings with him. The physician's task is to help the patient accept the reality of his situation, to help him make a realistic appraisal of it, to permit him the opportunity to voice his concerns, and to help him begin to deal constructively with the situation.

2 PLANNING TREATMENT

When more data must be gathered, by laboratory or radiological studies, for instance, the patient should be presented with a clear plan for future action. This will be discussed in detail later in this chapter.

When there is sufficient data and treatment can proceed, the physician's instructions should be equally clear and detailed. And it is quite important that the patient's involvement is such that "getting well" is the mutual aim of physician and patient. The patient, in other words, should share the physician's therapeutic goals, understand their respective roles in the treatment, and be prepared to be a responsible partner in the undertaking.

An approach some physicians use in attempting to motivate their patients is to frighten them into following their instructions carefully. This is always an error. Fear makes people less capable of listening and remembering. This was well-demonstrated by a study of fear-arousing communication,[3] in which a fifteen-minute illustrated lecture was prepared in three forms, all containing the same essential information about causes of tooth decay and the same recommendations about oral hygiene. One contained a very strong cautionary appeal emphasizing such unpleasant consequences of bad dental habits as pain, advanced gum disease, secondary illnesses, and ugly teeth; and it was made personal (that is, "*this* could happen to you"). The moderate appeal presented the same information less stridently and the minimal appeal rarely alluded to the consequences of tooth neglect. The subjects were divided into three groups, each of which heard one of the lectures. Their immediate and later responses were studied. The strong appeal aroused the greatest emotional response; however, the attitudes and oral hygiene practices of the group who heard the minimal appeal had changed within one week while neither changed in the strong appeal group. One year later a follow-up questionnaire indicated that conformity to the recommended practices was still significantly higher in the minimal than in the strong appeal group. There was evidence that the strong appeal had aroused fear and anger followed by a defensive avoidance of the internal and external cues that were present when the fear was aroused. In other words, frightening the subjects in the experiment had "turned them off."

It is better to take an educational approach. This means a clear and informative discussion in non-technical language of the treatment aims and the relationship of each part of the treatment plan to the treatment goals. Once it is clear that the patient understands and accepts the aims, the clinician can proceed with directions. But getting commitment from the patient to those aims is the most important single factor in assuring that he will follow directions.

To clarify whether the patient understands the treatment plan and is committed to it and to the goals of treatment, it is well for the physician to ask him to summarize what he will do. In order for the patient to restate the physician's recommendations he must understand them. The physician can reinforce them by writing them out for the patient.

3 SPECIAL PROBLEMS

"I Don't Know"

Probably the most difficult situation for both physician and patient is when the diagnosis, and consequently future treatment, is unclear. This may be the case because the total amount of information about the problem is inadequate, or because the physician's skill and knowledge are inadequate to make maximal use of the available information. In the first instance, more information may be sought. It may be, however, that the patient's problem has not evolved far enough in its biological course to reveal diagnostic clues; necessary information may not yet be available. In the second instance, a consultant with specialized skills and knowledge may be brought in.

It is important to clarify which of the two situations obtains in any instance, as they call for very different approaches. Though the liberal use of consultation has much to recommend it, except in those cases where consultation is urgently needed, problems may be created if it is called for too early—that is, before a firm doctor-patient relationship has been established. This may lead to a premature and inaccurate judgment about the physician's skills, and a good relationship of mutual trust and cooperation may never be reached. Lines of communication and areas of responsibility between primary physician, consultant, and patient may become confused. The patient's anxiety may be raised by the inference that consultation means a serious or life-threatening disease. And one must be reasonably certain that consultation will help, as it may be both expensive and futile if, in fact, the problem is undiagnosable.

As stated before, a clear plan for future action is called for when a diagnosis cannot yet be reached. This should include a direct admission, without evasiveness, that a diagnosis has not yet been made, a statement of what has been learned, and a description of the plan for observation and further study. If possible, an estimate should be given of the length of time required to make a definite diagnosis. If symptomatic therapy is to be carried on in the interval, its purpose (to control discomfort) should be stated. The primary objective of this discussion with the patient is to establish that he is not being abandoned, that the physician remains concerned, will see him regularly, and be alertly observant, and that the physician is prepared to act promptly when the situation changes.

If uncertainty persists for more than a few weeks, the patient will require increasing reassurance and support. Though the physician should indicate concern, it is important to avoid communicating anxiety to the patient. An unpublished study of a group of patients by Greene and Swisher indicated that major problems of patient management, including breakdown of the doctor-patient relationship and serious psychological distress in the patient or physician, occur more commonly in the situation of indeterminacy and indecision than in the management of the severely or fatally ill patient.

Referrals

If the physician decides that consultation is needed, he should discuss it with the patient. Preparation for a consultation is an important part of patient care, unfortunately omitted in far too many cases. Considerable anxiety in patients could be avoided if this matter were given more attention.

The referring physician should describe his reasons for requesting consultation, what procedures the patient will undergo, and what will follow. If it is clear that a number of visits to the consultant will be required, the physician should say so. Similarly, the referring physician should give the consultant a complete report of his findings and state his reasons for requesting consultation and what he expects from it.

Some delicacy is required in referring a patient to a psychiatrist for consultation or possible treatment. The patient may have a variety of fears and concerns and often a good deal of resistance to the idea. A single discussion with the patient may not be sufficient. After a tactful description of the reasons for the referral, it is important that the physician encourage the patient to express his concerns or questions and to deal with them factually but supportively. Frequent questions that arise are "Do you mean I'm imagining this?", "Does this mean I'm not really sick?", and "Do you think I'm mentally ill?" Making a successful referral in this case depends on taking enough time to deal with such questions and concerns.

"Do you think I'm imagining this?" calls for a firm and clear "No." This should be followed by a simple and non-technical explanation of the clinician's concept of the relationship between the evidences of psychological difficulties (such as anxiety, depression, or family conflicts, for example) and the symptoms experienced by the patient. Simple psychophysiological mechanisms can be described where appropriate, such as the relationship between anxiety and heart rate, or depression and general psychomotor retardation. Questions about mental illness require that the clinician find out what the patient's concept of mental illness is. When these are related to a memory of a senile relative or a psychotic family member, one is usually in a position to be honestly reassuring. Again, a description of the relationship between emotional conflict and its consequences on the one hand and physiological symptoms on the other can be helpful. When the reason for referral is that evidence from the interview and mental status examination indicate that the patient might be psychotic, tact is essential. "I think you do have mental and emotional problems, but I think Dr. B_____ may be able to help you" emphasizes the positive element of the potential for help in the consultation, rather than the labeling.

In some cases, more than one appointment with the patient may be necessary before the patient will accept a psychiatric referral.

Fatal Illness

When the findings indicate that there is a high probability that the patient is probably suffering from a fatal illness, the physician is likely to feel some conflict about how to discuss this. How much should he tell? Should the facts be presented to the patient, to the family, or to both?

The degree to which this will be a problem tends to vary with the diagnosis. Attitudes of physicians and patients differ toward the various kinds of fatal illness. Cancer or leukemia, for instance, carries with it the automatic expectation of a downhill course and slow painful death. A myocardial infarction in a patient with severe coronary arteriosclerosis has the same prognosis yet the patient will almost invariably feel more optimistic. He is likely to feel that death will be sudden. In the progressive respiratory insufficiency associated with severe pulmonary fibrosis the course will be progressively, inexorably downhill. Even so, it is not greeted with the degree of pessimism and despondency that attends the diagnosis of cancer, even though the future pain and suffering may be worse and the possibility of periods of remission far less.

Is it necessary to tell the patient that he is going to die? Not always. In the instance of malignancy, Kübler-Ross[4] feels that a doctor should speak freely with his patient about the diagnosis without equating it necessarily with impending death. He should leave the door open for hope (new drugs, treatments, new research findings) and, most important, that all is not lost, the patient will not be abandoned, and that patient, family, and doctor will fight together, whatever the end result.

At this point some, though by no means all, patients will ask, "How long do I have to live?" We agree with Kübler-Ross that the worst possible answer is to name a specific length of time. For one thing, it cannot be done with certainty. If the clinician names a specific length of time, whether the patient reaches a terminal stage before the predicted date, or survives beyond it, there will be problems for patient, family, and doctor. But another reason not to be specific is that this suggests a finality that can be devastating to the patient. All patients want to keep a door open to possible continued existence, however realistic they may be about their chances.

If the patient is under the age of ten, it is best not to introduce the topic of death. The diagnosis is given to the parents and the prognosis discussed with them. It should be described as ranges of time, the indeterminacy of the length of time stressed, and the support of the physician and health team stated and emphasized. On the other hand, one should not be evasive or tell untruths if a child who has a fatal disease asks questions. Here the principle is, tell no more than is asked. Tell it in simple words. Stress the fact that all possible care will be given and that there is hope. It may be appropriate to say more as the child approaches death and asks if he is going to die. But most young children have no concept of death and consider it to be something like going to sleep. One five-year-old child said to her mother, "Bury me in the back yard. Then when you die, you can be there too, and I'll reach out under the leaves and hold your hand."

With adults, the clinician should work toward an understanding of the situation at the rate chosen by the patient. This means answering questions honestly and making time available to the patient so that he may talk about his feelings and ask whatever questions he may have. One should never force information on a patient that he is not yet able to accept.

A knowledge of the patient's psychological and emotional makeup is essential in deciding how to tell and how much to tell. The patient who denies that he is fatally ill must be permitted time to accept the facts slowly, and if he cannot, should be permitted to deny them. The cool, objective, somewhat compulsive person may ask for a detailed scientific explanation. This should be given. Others want to know the bare mimimum, no more. This, too, should be respected. To choose the right approach one must know the patient.

In any event malignancy should never be presented as hopeless, with a "nothing can be done" tone. This will increase despondency and cause withdrawal, sometimes deep depression, and often rapid deterioration.

In some cultures, death is a greater blow to the family than to the patient. In those cultures where religious faith promises a life after death and family ties are very close, the patient may accept the knowledge of a fatal illness and impending death with equanimity, while the family may be quite upset and begin to mourn at once. In such cases, the physician should work with the family according to the very same principles, above, that he would use with the patient.

As death approaches, one can expect a series of changes in the patient's attitude toward himself, the world, and his approaching end of existence. Kübler-Ross[4] describes the responses of over two hundred patients at the University of Chicago Billings Hospital as going through five stages: denial and isolation, anger, bargaining, depression, and acceptance. At each stage, the interviewer's task is essentially the same: to listen to the patient, to tell him as much as he wants to hear, and to be supportive. The opportunity to talk should always be offered to the patient but never forced on him. The interviewer's non-verbal behavior, indicating his interest in listening, and a supportive attitude are most important.

Patients who achieve the state of acceptance die in peace and with dignity. Not all reach this stage, and there are patients who "fight" death with denial, alternating with anger or depression to the very end. The clinician should try to be available to talk with those patients with such responses and thus help them to achieve a state of acceptance. Good interviewing, permitting the widest range of possible topics to the patient to discuss, with help from the clinician in expressing feelings, followed by support and the opportunity to continue to talk about such feelings, will bring many patients to a state of acceptance.

Throughout the terminal care of the dying patient, attention must be given to his family. The family will undergo stages very similar to those of the patient and require similar help from the clinician if they, too, are to achieve a state of acceptance.

REFERENCES

1. Blum, R. H., *The Management of the Doctor-Patient Relationship*. New York: McGraw-Hill, 1960, p. 127.
2. Blum, R. H., Ibid., pp. 179-183.
3. Hovland, C. L., I. L. Janis, and H. H. Kelley, *Communication and Persuasion*. New Haven: Yale University Press, 1953.
4. Kübler-Ross, E., *On Death and Dying*. New York: The Macmillan Company, 1969.

10

THE SOCIAL CONTEXT OF THE CLINICAL INTERVIEW

Leta McKinney Adler, Ph.D.

1 INTRODUCTION

Much of this book has been concerned with ways to achieve the twin goals of the clinical interview: obtaining valid, reliable, and precise knowledge relevant to the patient's problems while at the same time promoting a helping relationship with the patient. The clinician has been described as the data gatherer, data processor and analyzer, decision maker and helper. It must not be forgotten, however, that the patient also processes and analyzes the communications he receives from the interviewer. He decides what information to offer, whether or not the interviewer's decisions are correct, and whether or not to follow the advice offered. In this chapter, the broader social context in which this communication and decision-making takes place will be examined.

Each patient and interviewer goes to the interview with certain expectations for his own and the other's behavior. They expect to fulfill the culturally defined roles of patient and professional as they understand them. Each takes his role differently depending not only on this understanding, but on his personal style of communication, family background, socio-economic status, and the ethnic, religious, and other subcultures in which he lives or has lived. The interview is also influenced by the physical setting and other aspects of the health care delivery system in which it occurs. All these factors may influence the choice an individual makes of the person to seek out for health care, the phase of illness in which he seeks help, the type of ailment for which he seeks help, his behavior in the interview, and his response to recommendations and treatment. Chapter 2 has already described some of the ways an individual's social background can affect his health status and health-care–seeking behavior.

2 THE PATIENT

In several earlier chapters we have described the effect of the patient's personality on the way he behaves in the interview. In Chapter 8 there was a discussion of the emotional responses of patients to illness and to the interviewer. It is also true that the patient's physical condition will affect his behavior. Nevertheless, it is possible to detect *patterns* of reciprocal behavior in most clinical interviews. These patterns are referred to by sociologists as reciprocal *role* behavior.

The Patient Role

The patient comes to the interview with preconceived ideas of what is expected of him, as well as of the behavior he expects of the clinician. These expectations, derived primarily from the general culture of the society in which he lives, are what behavioral scientists term the "social role of the patient." The patient's perception of this role may come from specific instruction in school or by his family, from his previous experience with physicians or other clinicians, from having observed the experiences of his relatives and friends with doctors, or through the portrayal of the doctor-patient relationship in movies, television, and literature. The patient role in our culture is strongly influenced by what health professionals view as appropriate behavior on the part of those seeking their help.

Social role is a concept used by behavioral scientists to describe the patterns of behavior shared by individuals occupying a certain position or fulfilling a certain function in a society. Our behavior varies to some extent according to the social context in which it occurs. We behave differently as we assume the roles of parent, husband, student, worker, poker player, and so on. Conversely, those with whom we interact respond to us differently depending on how they understand our appropriate role in a given social context. That is, they anticipate how we will behave in the social role they attribute to us and respond with this prediction in mind. The response of the other individual often represents a reciprocal role which we in our turn expect him to perform. Examples are the relationships between husband and wife, parent and child, salesman and customer, friend and friend. The roles of health care professionals and patients represent such reciprocal roles. All of these involve complementary expectations for the other's behavior.

Of course, individuals do not play social roles in the way that actors play dramatic roles, that is, by adhering to a script and doing exactly what is expected. Aside from the fact that each individual is unique, it is evident that knowing the expectations of another does not necessarily result in conforming to those expectations. Conformity usually occurs when both parties to the interaction believe that their individual goals may thus be met. In other situations, such as those in which an individual does not share the goal of the other or distrusts the other, he is very likely to assess the behavior of the other and to respond cautiously or not at all in the way expected. For example, a distrustful individual might behave with his doctor in a way that reflects his belief that he must be on guard against exploitation or ineptitude. The involuntary psychiatric patient and some children brought to the clinical situation for the first time will behave in this way, since they and the clinician do not share a common goal. Goffman[1] has termed this type of behavior "strategic interaction."

To some extent, the interviewer always behaves as if the interview were a strategic interaction since he knows that the patient does not share his scientific knowledge and thus, through ignorance, cannot totally share the goal of developing *relevant* information. He may also engage in strategic interaction under other circumstances, for example, when he suspects that the patient is malingering; is providing false, biased, or inaccurate information; is deceiving the physician with respect to his compliance with the treatment plan, or when he wishes to persuade the patient of the efficacy of a treatment which the patient rejects. Some patients (and some professionals) are more inclined to distrust than others; the "paranoid personality" habitually engages in strategic interaction.

The patient usually assumes a sick role before he adopts a patient role. The sick role may be thought of as a deviant role since it prevents the individual from fulfilling some or all of his socially defined functions. This deviant role, however, is usually not morally condemned if it is assumed under the following conditions: First, the incapacity of the individual is considered impossible to overcome by an act of will on his part. Second the sick person recognizes his deviant state and exhibits a "desire to get well" and to return to social functioning within the limits of his capacity. And finally, he expresses this desire by consulting and following the recommendations of a health authority deemed appropriate by others in his social setting. When the incapacity is viewed as caused by the sick person, perhaps through his failure to "take care of himself," he is not accorded exemption from disapproval and often suffers guilt and remorse.[2] This circumstance does not exempt him from the remaining requirements of the sick role; indeed, strict adherence to the treatment regime may serve as kind of an "expiation" of the "sin" committed against his health.

It is the last aspect of the sick role that brings the patient to the attention of the health professional and forms the core of the patient role. In present-day American society, the physician is generally considered to be the most appropriate person to consult; however, for minor illnesses a family member or neighbor may suffice. In some subcultures, the advice of a folk healer may be sought first. The pharmacist at the corner drug store may be consulted, as may a wide variety of other sources of care, such as chiropractors and faith healers. As the team concept of health care gains ground, the patient will increasingly come into contact with a variety of health professionals. More and more often, the principal clinician encountered by the patient will be a nurse, social worker, health technician, or an assistant to the physician.

The patient role has been socially defined primarily in relation to the reciprocal role of physician. Much of what has been written applies to the patient role in relation to other health professionals. There is some evidence, however, that the patient's role expectations for himself and the interviewer are somewhat different when other health professionals conduct the interview. These differences will be considered later in this chapter.

Acceptable role behavior requires of the patient that he "put himself in the hands" of the physician and exhibit "a desire to get well." The patient's behavior will reflect his acceptance of the doctor's authority and his willingness to surrender some of his autonomy. Accordingly, he is usually somewhat passive. He may volunteer information only as encouraged by the doctor to do so, and he may attempt to restrict the information he gives to the general area about which the physician indicates he is interested. The patient is also likely to do whatever he can to keep the level of tension low, that is, to please the doctor. One of the important consequences of the role behavior of patients is the reciprocal effect that the physician may inadvertently cut off communication by exerting too much authority and by requesting only highly specific information.

The patient will come prepared to speak more freely about his body, his discomforts, and his pain than in other social situations and he will be more reserved in speaking of aspects of life which he considers unrelated to health and illness. Since the patient's role includes compliance with the physician's authority, the patient is usually prepared to accept the doctor's definitions of what is relevant to health and illness and to modify his behavior to meet the physician's expectations.

The Patient's Culture and Socio-economic Status

The conditions under which an individual assumes the sick role and the way in which he performs the patient role vary greatly with the culture and subcultures in which he participates as well as with his socio-economic class. The sick role and the patient role as defined above are descriptions which most accurately fit white, urban, educated, middle- and upper-class, old-stock Americans. It is individuals of this background whose definitions of health and illness are most congruent with those of the health professional. These are the individuals whose conditions of life permit exemption from social responsibilities because of illness. They are most likely to take an optimistic view of the probable outcome of the medical care, having most frequently experienced this, and to have faith in science as an instrument of change. Thus it is individuals of this background who are most likely to visit the doctor in the phase of illness and for the conditions the doctor considers appropriate. They are also most likely to fulfill the patient role in a way that meets the expectations of the clinician. They are most likely to "follow the doctor's orders" and permit lengthy, costly, or uncomfortable treatment procedures in the expectation of improved health.

In contrast, the Mexican-Americans of the Santa Clara Valley in California are reported by Clark[3] to resist the sick role and the patient role because these roles do not exempt the individual from deviant status. Barrio people fear that their family and friends will somehow lose respect for them, that they will be considered "different" or "inferior." An individual who begins to feel ill makes every effort to continue his regular activities. He gets social approval not by "taking care of himself" and seeking early medical attention but by ignoring illness as long as possible. Men of the barrio particularly resist succumbing to illness, not only because the consequences for an hourly wage worker are economically disastrous but because illness is not *macho*, or ruggedly masculine. In addition, illness is viewed fatalistically as not under the control of the patient. Where middle-class Anglos tend to blame themselves for illness, attributing it to negligence or poor health habits, the Mexican-American tends to blame external forces, sometimes including witches and evil spirits. He blames himself only for "giving in" too soon by consulting a physician. For many conditions, he will consult a *curandero,* or folk healer, first. From the standpoint of the physician, such a patient frequently consults him too late.

Other instances of cultural and socio-economic differences and their influence on health care seeking and interview behavior are discussed in Chapter 2.

The Patient's Family

Usually, it is in his family that a patient is defined as ill, and it is there that the sick role is first adopted. It is usually within the family that the decision is made to consult a health authority and the one to be consulted is selected. As indicated above, these decisions are strongly influenced by socio-economic and cultural factors. In many instances, the illness of the patient is itself a reflection of disturbances in the family.

In the days when much medical care took place in the home, the physician was able to make direct observations of the family's life style, the patient's role in his family and the complex interrelationships among family members, and to assess their effect on the one he was examining. These are not so obvious when an interview takes place in the doctor's office or a hospital.

Not only has the location of medical care changed, but the patterm of family life has changed since the days when the family doctor made the rounds of his patients' homes with his horse and buggy or Model-T. At that time the *nuclear family*—that is, husband, wife, and their unmarried children—often was embedded in the *extended family,* a kinship group which might include grandparents, married brothers and sisters, their spouses and children, as well as aunts, uncles, and other relatives. The household often included relatives other than members of the nuclear family, and related nuclear families often lived close to each other. This pattern prevailed not only in rural areas, but in cities, where residents frequently had migrated from rural areas of this country or of countries abroad. Some Italian-American and Greek-American families in eastern seaboard cities and Mexican-American families in southwestern cities still continue this family pattern. In these families the clinician must work with the whole family in order to be effective with the patient.

The extended family provided relationships that were mutually supportive, both economically and emotionally. Decision-making was shared, and in times of crisis, such as illness, there was a great deal of immediately available help and emotional support. Child care was shared by a number of adults and sickness of a parent did not mean that a child would be deprived of love and parental care, as another adult well known to the child could move into the parental role instantly.

But the extended family has become less significant in American life. With most workers now dependent on the labor market, the nuclear family must be mobile and live wherever the wage-earner finds a job. Thus, for most Americans today, the kinship ties of the extended family have been loosened. The nuclear family, smaller than it once was, now tends to live alone, often far away from others in the extended family.

The functions performed by the family have likewise changed. When the family was a producing unit, the work of women and children was required to produce many goods and services for the household. Now the primary economic function of the family is to serve as a consumption unit. The work still done in the home is largely mechanized and automated so that little labor is required. All of this means that the economic bonds which used to bind family members are much weaker. The clear definition of family roles around tasks to be performed is gone; family stability is reduced. The extended family pattern of mutual help is frequently burdensome where it survives. Maiden aunts or ailing brothers-in-law, are now just one more mouth for the wage-earner to feed and increase the crowding in his small urban dwelling unit. Responsibilities to extended family members may drive all below the poverty level.

As the economic functions of the family declined and the bonds of the extended family loosened, modern urbanized, industrialized society grew more impersonal and anonymous. The individual's social relations outside the family became more fragmented. Consequently, the already weakened, nuclear family has become the chief source of emotional support and intimacy for its members. The provision of intimate, supportive relationships is now the chief function of the nuclear family, aside from the physical care and socialization of young children. Its ability to do so may be severely taxed by illness of one of its members.

With these changes in family function and structure, family roles have also changed. The husband-father is usually away at work all day. The wife-mother typically remains at home, at least before the children enter school. She cares for the children and performs household tasks. The maintenance of the health of family members and the care of sick members is part of this wife-mother role. The mother also carries most of the burden of providing love, warmth, and support to family members. The husband-father in higher status families shares this function more frequently than in working-class or lower-class families.

The husband-father is typically the chief provider and usually the principal authority figure in the family. The lower the class status of the father, the greater the difficulty he tends to have in maintaining his decision-making position, which derives from the respect of other family members, which is influenced by his success as a provider. On the other hand, the upper-class father is likely to share his authority with his wife. In this class, the democratic family ideal often leads to the sharing of significant decision-making with the children.

The family as described above, with its class-related variations, represents the modal pattern in the United States. However, as is true of all intimate relationships and groups, each family is to some extent unique because of the individuality of its members. Expressive and authority roles may be reversed, or one parent may be the more important in fulfilling both roles. The lower-class family is frequently matriarchal in form. Discipline of children varies among families and is thought to be more consistent and more oriented toward cultivation of valued personality traits in the upper classes than in the lower classes, where the struggle to provide food, clothing, and shelter for the children is of necessity the overriding consideration. The above description of the family also focussed on one phase of the family life cycle. The period before children enter the family and the "empty-nest" period have different characteristics, an increasingly important feature being the employment of the wife outside the home.

It also must not be forgotten that many American families in the child-rearing period are one-parent families, most frequently fatherless families. This means that one parent must attempt to fulfill both authority and expressive functions. This probably does not present an insurmountable obstacle to family functioning though the consequences of the one-parent family for the socialization of children are not well understood. Lastly, it must not be forgotten that many individuals do not live in family groups. In urban areas, many live alone or with roommates.

In Chapters 7 and 8, the interviewing of a child and his parent and the interviewing of the patient's family have been discussed. Such interviews offer the clinician an opportunity to observe at first hand the relationships among family members. Nevertheless, he should not forget that he is observing the family in only one situation. If the wife-mother dominates the conversation, he should not necessarily conclude that she dominates all aspects of family life; she may be assuming her role as chief provider and supervisor of health care in her family. Conversely, a husband-father might not sit by passively in other situations which he regards as requiring him to act in his own family role, such as the purchase of life insurance. The interviewer should be observant of all family members, not simply the one designated as patient. In cases of psychiatric illness, it has often been observed that the most disturbed individual family member is not always selected by the family as the patient. The family interview will also give the interviewer an opportunity to assess the importance of disturbed family relationships in the physical illness of the patient, coupled with what the patient reports in private to the clinician.

One purpose of this discussion is to highlight the variety in family functions, roles, and norms. The interviewer should be aware that family function, to be effective, need not conform to his own values for marriage and family life. He should also be aware that an assessment of the patient's family, its way of functioning, and its stability is important in diagnosis, as well as in planning treatment for most patients.

3 THE INTERVIEWER

Like the patient, the interviewer's behavior in conducting the interview is in many respects a product of his history, his own subcultural reference groups, and his social role. Personal characteristics, including the way he has learned to handle authority throughout his life, will influence his behavior as well as how he and the patient relate to each other. He will tend to behave with the patient as authority figures in his life have behaved. His behavior with patients will also reflect the way he has learned to deal with others who were subordinate, weaker, or more helpless than he, such as younger brothers and sisters and younger friends. He may have learned to give help to those of lower status in a way that shows respect for their need to feel self-esteem or in an uninvolved, didactic, dogmatic, authoritarian, or even contemptuous manner which robs the individual being assisted of his independence, self-confidence, or self-esteem. There are technique-oriented physicians and nurses who value procedures and skilful handling of instruments more than the feelings of the patient. Diagnosis and treatment are challenges to the intellectual and technical skills of such physicians. Person-oriented health professionals see their role more clearly as the relief of suffering. Each of these two contrasting orientations has its social value. However, extremes in each—the cold and highly impersonal professional on the one hand and the over-involved professional who undertakes to "rescue" patients from every difficulty, on the other—can interfere with good communication and reduce the amount and accuracy of important information in the interview. The first fails to deal with significant psychosocial aspects of illness and the second fosters over-dependence or unrealistic expectations for the relationship.

The Professional Role

Unlike the patient, the interviewer has been trained to subject much of his personal behavior to the professional discipline which governs his conduct in the interview. The medical student, for example, undergoes a long and rigorous socialization process which inculcates in him the appropriate role behavior for a physician in our society. This role includes not only technical skills but a variety of prescribed and proscribed behaviors defining the nature of his relationship to his patients. Other health professionals are subject to similar, though usually less intensive, socialization. To clarify this socialization of personal behavior, it is helpful to examine the health professional's role in the light of sociological studies of professions.

A profession consists of a set of roles that shape behavior toward professional colleagues and other persons in the work situation, as well as toward individuals receiving professional services. His profession is usually of such significance to the professional person that it influences his conduct in many social situations where he is not acting in a professional capacity. The professional role may be viewed as consisting of three types of behavior: instrumental activities, which are the skills and procedures by which professional work is accomplished; expressive activities, which create the emotional climate in which the professional work is carried out; and control activities, in which decisions are initiated or made for others. It is in the interview that the health professional's role is established.

Medicine, perhaps more than any other field, fits the model of a profession. In fact, this model was constructed primarily by sociological investigation of medicine. Thus, the physician's professional role is one of the best documented of all occupational roles and it is the standard against which the degree of "professionalization" of other occupations is likely to be assessed. The consideration of the doctor's role is therefore of consequence to all health professionals.

The characteristics of a profession have been variously enumerated.[4, 5, 6, 7, 8] In the following, the implications for the interview of four major characteristics usually attributed to a professional role are described with special reference to the physician.

1. A profession possesses a complex body of special knowledge concerning significant and difficult tasks and enjoys a publicly sanctioned monopoly of this knowledge. Professional knowledge is acquired by lengthy training supervised by members of the profession. In the case of the health professions and certain others, it is subject to examination and licensing procedures carried out by the profession with the authority of the state. The monopolistic character attributed to professional knowledge creates strong pressure on the patient to accept a subordinate role in the interview, since he has need of information or skills to which he may gain access only through a member of the profession. For the same reason, the patient's dependence is accepted and, under some circumstances, legitimately encouraged.

The authority of the physician and the importance of the doctor-patient relationship is enhanced in the eyes of the layman by the special quality of medical knowledge. It embraces the most mysterious and significant aspects of human existence, birth, and death. Furthermore, of the three traditional established professions (medicine, law, and theology), medicine is the only one to base its practice on scientific research, giving it the added prestige of science. There are elements in the respect with which medicine is regarded that border on the sacredness in which the priesthood is held.

An important element in the development of a patient's trust in the physician is the patient's evaluation of his competence, that is, his mastery of professional knowledge. Successful treatment is, of course, an important way of establishing competence in the eyes of the patient. Another is skill in using certain techniques, procedures, and instruments, a highly visible part of the physician's role. Beyond their specific function his use of these skills and technical "hardware" have an effect on the doctor-patient relationship. They identify the doctor to the patient as a skilled technician thus enhancing the basis of his authority. Physicians whose offices and personal conduct overemphasize medical hardware and technical procedures may, however, be attempting to use the prestige of "science" to maintain the patient's confidence.

2. The public believes and demands that members of a profession display a higher degree of, and a more selfless, involvement in their occupation and the services they provide than is characteristic of non-professional occupations. This second characteristic implies the loyalty of the physician to his patient, including the well-known professional ethic of confidentiality. It is because the definition of a profession includes this notion of "avowal,"[9] that the professional receives and expects a higher level of trust from those he serves than other producers of goods and services receive. It is this aspect of the physician's role that encourages the patient to speak freely about private matters in the interview and, together with his judgment of the physician's technical competence, to cooperate with the treatment plan.

The role of the doctor, more than that of other major professions, includes an expectation that services will be rendered in a warm, sympathetic, understanding, and often "fatherly" (or "motherly") manner. The physician meets this expectation for his behavior in the interview through attentiveness to the patient's communication and a genuine display of interest in helping the patient with his problems. When the patient's expectations for considerate, sympathetic help are not met, he is often deeply disappointed or angry. Because of the public's high expectations for the physician's enactment of his professional role, laymen feel outraged when they believe that an individual doctor, or doctors collectively, place monetary or other personal rewards and satisfactions above humanitarian concerns.

3. The professional person maintains a degree of emotional neu-

trality toward those he serves. This quality of the professional role sets limits on the extent of personal involvement expected by the patient from the physician. It preserves the clinician's own emotional balance and personal life. It also serves the patient by assuring him that personal involvement will not impair the physician's judgment. The custom that doctors do not treat their own families testifies to the dangers inherent in treating a patient with whom one is emotionally and personally involved. Most patients understand this aspect of the doctor's role. There are those, however, who wish for a personal rather than a professional relationship. They will tend to scrutinize the actions of the physician for signs in his behavior that can nourish their fantasies. Thus, in order not to encourage unrealistic expectations which lead to a troubled doctor-patient relationship it is incumbent upon the physician to preserve this aspect of his role both inwardly and outwardly.

4. A professional is organized, autonomous, and self-regulating. The individual professional is loyal to his profession and to his colleagues. His work is rarely subject to evaluation and regulation by others. Evaluation by his peers means that all aspects of a physician's practice, including his interview behavior, will be strongly influenced by the medical community in which he works and by his professional affiliations. Through medical schools, state licensing and regulatory bodies, county medical societies, speciality boards, and hospital staff organizations, the physician's professional (and even non-professional) behavior is regulated and controlled by other physicians.

The values and standards of the local medical community will influence the doctor's behavior with his patients to a very significant degree. There is a tendency in every medical community to conform with regard to favored drugs, patterns of referral, attitudes toward mental illness, etc. One study indicated that this conformity is so great that in order to influence a medical community to adopt a new practice or change an attitude, it is necessary to identify trend-setters, or innovators, who are willing to try something new and persuade them to make a change. Only then will it be adopted, first by a small group called "early adopters." Finally, the bulk of the group of physicians, the "late adopters," will shift to the new practice thus preserving conformity.[10]

The regulating influence of the medical community is increased in its effectiveness by the fact that a medical community is really a network of interconnecting small groups and "stimuli that impinge on any member of the community set in motion processes that will, with varying degrees of speed and thoroughness, pervade the rest of the community" as Coleman and his co-workers have phrased it.[11] These networks include hospital attending staff associations, office partnerships and clinics, informal discussion at lunch or in the staff lounge or cloakroom of the community hospital. Social friendships are also important to this regulative network since doctors tend to socialize chiefly with each other after hours.

Challenges to medical self-regulation are increasingly making their appearance, however. The frequency of malpractice suits has been increasing for many years and the legal definition of malpractice is changing. Non-physician administrators of hospitals and clinics exert increasingly important indirect influence in the practice of physicians. The physician's autonomy in treating the patient is being diminished by the growth of other health professions with their own demands for professional autonomy based on their specialized knowledge as well as the fact that they share more and more of the physician's formerly exclusive knowledge. The interests of third-party payers in some cases affect the manner in which the physician practices. The planning and operation of publicly supported medical facilities are increasingly influenced by citizen's groups, often the consumers of the health services being provided.

The salaried physician may be subject to control by his employer over at least some aspects of the practice of his profession. Of course, it should not be overlooked that the private, fee-for-service practitioner has always been subtly controlled by his patients, except in communities where there is a shortage of physicians. He must please his patients sufficiently to maintain a practice, and the nature of his patients' complaints determine the professional skills he will exercise. His mobility is always less than that of a salaried professional because of the necessity to reestablish a practice in a new locale.

The physician's professional role, including his relative freedom to perform his work without supervision from outside his profession, his position as an arm of the law, for example, with respect to psychiatric and infectious diseases, and the profession's success in enlisting the state to enforce professional standards, enhances the authority of the physician in the interview and influences his behavior accordingly.

The Nurse's Role

Hospital nurses and office nurses usually do not practice autonomously, though the time is long past when the nurse rose as the doctor approached the nursing station or deferred to him as they entered an elevator. This is largely because much of the knowledge used by nurses is medical, that is, knowledge over which physicians exert final authority. Yet, subordination of the nurse to the physician often creates difficulties in communication between the nurse and both the physician and "his" patient. She is often called upon to exert extreme tact with the former and evasive tactics with the latter. She may be discouraged from reporting valuable observations about the patient to that physician who emphasizes his superior status. Usually she does not feel free to deal with the patient's questions or worries about prognosis, medications, and so forth, even though it might be therapeutic if she were to respond to the patient's feelings when he has the courage to voice them.

Nursing, more than any other role within the health professions, is defined as belonging to women.[12] Thus, part of the nurse's subordination to physicians, who are mostly male in the United States, is a reflection of traditional sex roles in our culture. Like women's role in our society, however, the role of nurse is changing as well.

With respect to other aspects of the professional role, the nurse's professionalization is well established. Altruistic motives have always been attributed to the nurse, and patients have well-defined expectations for her warmth and care. Nurses have also usually been trained to temper emotional involvement with professional objectivity though their socialization into this aspect of their professional role may not be as intensive as for physicians or social workers.

The majority of nurses practice in hospitals and most of what has been written about the nurse's role concerns the hospital nurse. Hospital patients expect a level of professional involvement from the nurse similar to that of the doctor. However, they probably look for a greater degree of warmth and psychological support from the nurse than from the doctor. Patients are more likely to excuse the actions of a gruff physician than similar ones on the part of a nurse. A cranky nurse usually produces a feeling of disappointment and outrage in the patient. These expectations on the part of patients are partly related to the fact that nurses are almost always women, partly to the traditional "Angel of Mercy" image of the nurse. To a great extent it is related to the nurse's view of her own role and to the way she tends to behave toward the patient.

Schulman[13] has described the modern nurse in terms of two basic functional roles: mother surrogate and healer. It is his view that the expressive aspects of the nurse role should approximate the mother's role toward her child. He describes the "mother surrogate" aspects of the nurse role as affectionate and intimate. It is characterized by physical proximity, which is greatest at the onset and least at the terminal phase of the relationship; orientation toward meeting the general needs of a dependent ward; and identification and protection of such a ward. He cites evidence that nurses see their role as having this component.

When a patient becomes seriously ill, he tends to regress emotionally, and he is very likely to see the nurse as just such a mother figure—comforting, protecting, and supporting—if he encounters her in the hospital setting, where most nurse-patient interviews take place. He is, therefore, likely to confide easily in the nurse who meets these expectations, to seek comfort from her actively and to accept dependency more easily than he might under ordinary circumstances. Very often, significant information about emotional problems or psychological aspects of the illness which could be obtained by the doctor only with difficulty, if at all, is easily obtained by the nurse.

Schulman's "mother surrogate" model for the nurse's expressive behavior must be viewed with some reservations. In the first place, it must be examined with respect to its effect on the patient. In an interview in which motherly behavior predominates, there is a greater danger of fostering dependency and regression than there is in more emotionally neutral interview situations. Furthermore, in the hospital situation, there is always the possibility of the patient becoming overly attached to the nurse and perhaps of misinterpreting the mother surrogate aspects of the nurse's behavior as a personal or romantic attachment to him. For this reason, the same professional reserve that characterizes the doctor's preferred role behavior should be maintained by the nurse. King[14] calls it controlled involvement or detached concern.

In the second place, the frequency of "mother surrogate" behavior in the actual activities of nurses is open to question. It is becoming more common that the expectations of the hospital patient for this warm, concerned care are not met. In any case, this view of the nurse's expressive behavior applies only to that bedside nurse whose personality enables her to function in this manner.

The Medical Social Worker's Role

Medical social work began in Boston in 1905 because of a growing awareness that social factors were an important part of disease and its treatment. The description of the medical social worker's role in the health team offered by H. H. Margolis in 1946 still holds true.

"In order to insure integrated help for the patient, the physician shares professional thinking and planning with the worker. We depend on her largely for an objective picture of the patient's social setting, his relationship with the family group, its socioeconomic as well as its emotional resources. . . . We see her as having capacity for helping the patient to participate more fully and comfortably in the doctor-patient relationship and in the processes of medical diagnosis and treatment. From her must come the specialized knowledge of community resources for vocational job placement and for meeting the other social needs of the patient related to his illness."[15]

Though regarded as subordinate to the physician, social workers generally have less difficulty than do nurses in asserting their professional status and achieving a degree of autonomy over their activities. Social workers have a body of knowledge and practice distinct from that of the physician. This knowledge and its clinical application is acquired in training at the graduate level, while a registered nurse frequently lacks even a baccalaureate degree. Furthermore, social work is practiced autonomously in non-medical settings, and it is not a distinctively female occupation, though women predominate in the field.

An obvious difference between the role of the social worker and those of the physician and nurse is the absence of physical procedures involving touching the patient or the use of instruments. This eliminates extreme physical intimacy and reduces the mystery in the relationship between the medical social worker and the patient. The patient is able to maintain more of his "well" identity with the social worker. This in itself helps him to overcome the regressive tendencies associated with illness and bed care as well as to maintain his self-concept and his self-esteem. On the other hand, not being in constant attendance upon the patient as is the nurse, the social worker is in a position to be more accepting of dependence and more tolerant of the overly demanding patient than nursing personnel. In addition, medical treatment, especially in the hospital, often requires passive acceptance of procedures administered by the physician or nurse whereas the social worker's professional services seldom require such passivity.

While the factors mentioned above, in themselves encourage self-determination and the maintenance of the patient's customary self-concept, such participation in the relationship is also an important goal of medical social work. According to one medical social worker, Minna Field, "particularly in dealing with those whose illness and incapacity tend to undermine their feelings of worth and status, the primary prerequisite is an appreciation of the worth and dignity of the individual and a respect for his rights as a human being, regardless of the stage of his illness or the degree of his impairment."[16] One social work textbook states that medical social work interviews "are directed toward action on the part of the patient in making the accommodation to the limitations of illness or the step toward health." This, the text continues, is accomplished when the social worker permits the patient to express his fears, takes him for what he is, instills confidence in him, thinks out some of his difficulties with him, and is available to work out further plans with him.[17] Thus the patient is likely to be more active, and the social worker to rely much less on her authority than the physician or nurse.

The most frequently utilized social work service in the medical setting is social casework, and the crucial element in casework is the interview. It is through the interview that the social worker achieves the goals listed above. The medical social worker is most often the member of the health team who works with the patient's family. The patient's family is interviewed not only to gain information which will assist in understanding the patient's illness and in developing a management plan appropriate to the family situation, but beyond that, in order to assist the family itself to meet the difficulties arising out of the illness of one of its members.

The medical social worker usually sees the patient upon referral from a physician or nurse who believes that some environmental situation is detrimental to the patient or that community resources outside the medical setting should be mobilized to assist the patient in some way. In certain health care organizations, social workers see patients routinely, rather than on referral. In modifying or mobilizing the patient's social environment, the social worker is frequently a "boundary worker" representing the hospital (or other medical care system) to other social organizations. This position at the interface between one organization and others is frequently a stressful one.[18] Sometimes the social worker functions as an intermediary between the patient and the health care system, interpreting the latter to the patient and mobilizing the system more effectively around the individual needs of a patient. In performing all these functions, the medical social worker's primary instrument is the interview.

The Interviewer's Socio-economic Status and Cultural Background

The clinician's behavior, like the patient's, is shaped by the shared values, beliefs, and attitudes that characterize the subcultures in which he lives and has lived. Some aspects of his behavior, such as his interest in patient's families, reflect as much of his cultural origins as his professional training. The family in which he grew up and his present family situation also influence his behavior directly and indirectly, as does his socio-economic status.

A great deal of sociological interest has been focused on the effects of class-status differences between the health professional and the patient. The physician in our society enjoys extremely high status. Although there is some evidence that the pattern is changing, physicians in the past have been recruited mainly from the upper and middle classes. Even when this is not the case, a physician achieves status through his profession. To a lesser degree the same may be said of social workers and nurses.

The physician and his high status patients agree most readily on the nature and appropriate response to illness. These patients, by virtue of a social status similar to the physician's, greater sophistication in matters of health, and their high standards for "wellness" are often less passive and submissive in the interview. They are frequently able to offer much of the required information spontaneously if permitted to do so by the interviewer. They are also less likely to be submissive in the doctor-patient relationship, and physicians frequently accept or promote a more equalitarian relationship with patients of equal social status.

Conversely, the interviewer may be misled by a lower-class patient's deference toward him as a high status person. Outward compliance or even subservience may hide a distrust of the physician, disbelief in scientific medicine, or unwillingness or inability to follow the recommended management plan. To a lesser extent nurses, social workers, and other health professionals experience the same social distance between themselves and many of their patients. The distrust of established medicine on the part of ghetto and barrio dwellers is based on class and ethnic differences in large measure. This distrust has prevented some from seeking needed medical care. The so-called "indigenous" health worker or health aide has been created to act as an intermediary between them and the professional health care system.

The possible ill effects on the interview of status difference between patient and interviewer have been described by Simmons. He has commented on the disparity between the ideal doctor's role as it interacts with the role of the patient and the reality of most doctor-patient relationships. Ideally, the doctor's role in the therapeutic relationship focuses on his performance of a technical specialty, on his impartiality in serving the patient's health needs independently of whether he likes the patient as a person, and on his obligation to give priority to the patient's well-being over his own personal interest. Simmons feels that this ideal role definition holds across the board in most Western societies though not in many non-Western societies. It is calculated to inspire trust, respect, and confidence between doctor and patient and thus to ensure cooperation. In practice, however, it seems that the ideal is seldom approximated in professional-patient relationships, and that it is precisely in the doctor-patient relationship where it is least likely to be achieved.

"Studies in intracultural situations, both here and in other societies, indicate a tendency for class considerations to overshadow therapeutic considerations in the professional-patient relationship. It appears that the degree to which the qualities ideally defined as essential to the therapeutic relationship, namely, mutual trust, respect, and cooperation, will be present in a given professional-patient relationship varies inversely with the amount of social distance. Conversely, the greater the social distance, the less likely that participants will perceive each other in terms of the ideal type roles of professional and patient, and the more likely that they will perceive each other in terms of their social status in the larger society."[19]

There is evidence that in the public health situation, patients and nurses "get along" better than patients and the higher status doctors.[20]

4 THE HEALTH CARE ORGANIZATION: THE INTERVIEW SETTING

The social systems discussed up to this point are primarily indirect influences on the interview through the behavior of the participants. Sometimes events in other systems produce psychological responses and states which are expressed in the interview. For example, the physician troubled by occurrences in his own family may be brusque or inattentive during the interview. Occasionally these extra-interview systems impinge directly on the interview as when the interviewer receives an emergency call from his home or when the patient's family is present. But it is the health care delivery system in which the interview takes place that affects the interview most directly. Both its organizational and physical characteristics influence the quality of the interview.

We may speak of any specific organization which delivers health care, such as a hospital, clinic, or physician's office, as a health care delivery system, or we may designate all the resources for health care, including preventive, diagnostic, therapeutic, and rehabilitative services, available to physicians and consumers in the community as constituting a health care delivery system. Some of these services unfortunately are frequently at some distance from most communities. Usually there are more or less distinct but somewhat overlapping health care delivery systems in a community. Usually there is a system offered by private physicians and voluntary hospitals to those who can afford it, on the one hand, and the various loosely organized health care services offered to the medically indigent by public agencies on the other. There may also be large group practices financed through pre-payment plans offering comprehensive health care to a large block of the employed population, and the federal government may offer what amounts to a parallel system for certain segments of the population. Some communities may also have university-connected medical centers which offer comprehensive health services or variously funded independent clinics.

There are two major, and interrelated, problems in the organization of health services, leaving aside the important issues of financing and ultimate control. One is the difficulty presently encountered in the provision of coordinated and comprehensive health care to the patient and the second is the alienating quality of modern medical care. Both have a direct effect on the interview.

Ideally, it is envisioned in the United States that all health care should be coordinated by a personal or family physician who would provide continuity in the health-maintaining and health-restoring care received by the patient. In addition, comprehensive care would be ensured. This physician himself would be the point of entry into the health care system. He would provide much of this care in his office; he would follow the patient into the hospital; and he would refer the patient to other medical specialists or to community resources as he deemed such referrals appropriate.

At the present time, even in the private health care delivery system this type of medical care is rarely received. It is provided, in varying degrees, to those who prefer and can afford it, by general practitioners, pediatricians, internists, and, occasionally, other medical specialists. Some other health care delivery systems endeavor with varying success to provide the equivalent of the "family doctor." In some neighborhood health centers, patients are assigned to a health team. In public systems, on the other hand, it may be unusual for a single physician to coordinate the care of a patient through one episode of illness. Often, each interview is a new encounter and requires a complete new data base.

The private physician conducts most extensive medical interviews in his office, his most congenial environment. It is here that he feels most at home and where, consequently, his most spontaneous behavior is likely to occur. Both the doctor's and the patient's behavior will be influenced by the way the office is used. Both can communicate more freely if the setting of the interview is a quiet consulting room with reasonably comfortable furniture and if there are few or no interruptions. While it is perhaps easiest to secure the conditions for a successful interview in the physician's office, it does not necessarily follow that these conditions will exist. Many physicians permit the telephone and office personnel to interrupt their interviews, do not allow sufficient time for the interview, or narrowly limit the topics discussed. Some physicians make a practice of conducting interviews in their examining rooms, where the patient is partially clothed or under a drape sheet on the examining table. The patient rarely feels at ease under such circumstances. He is likely to feel both powerless and self-estranged without the clothing which announces his identity to others and confirms it for himself. The social distance between the doctor and the patient is likely to be increased. Docility, obedience, embarrassment, and efforts to please the physician will reduce the amount of information from the patient and sometimes bias it.

The least suitable setting for the outpatient interview is probably the clinic of a large public hospital. The physical setting is likely to be uncomfortable and unattractive and it is likely to afford little privacy. The physician is usually on a tight time schedule. Both the physician and the patient are likely to be caught in a maze of bureaucratic procedures and frequently both are aware that the patient will see a different physician on his next clinic visit. Usually the interview brings together a doctor and patient of quite different socio-cultural backgrounds with the many attending difficulties. All of these create problems that require a great effort on the part of the physician and the other health workers, if they are to be overcome. While it will probably require a major organizational overhaul to provide comprehensive, coordinated patient care in municipal health care systems, an effective interview on the part of a clinic physician can go a long way toward providing the basis for such care to the patients he sees.

Alienative Features of Health Care

Alienation refers to feelings of disconnectedness from, and disenchantment with, one's society and its organizations, values, and norms (or standards). Sociologists identify four facets of alienation: feelings of powerlessness, normlessness, meaninglessness, and self-estrangement. One of the reasons for the alienating quality of health care is lack of continuity and coordination in the highly specialized health services received by patients. They are frequently made to feel not only that they are overlooked as a person or viewed only as a human body but that they are regarded as a set of organ systems, each in the hands of a different medical specialty. The interface between the patient and the health care system is the interview, and it is almost decisive in determining whether these problems will be overcome in the patients' treatment.

Seeman and Evans[21] state that medical care "represents a microcosm of the alienative features" of mass society in that it is a situation with "low control over one's fate, heavy reliance upon specialized experts, bureaucratic authority, and the loss of community ties."

The patient may feel alienated in the hands of private physicians in those situations, far too common, where he must suffer long periods of waiting in reception areas and examining rooms, where he may be under treatment simultaneously by four or five medical specialists whose communication is faulty if not altogether absent, where he may understand little of what is done to him and where he must wait days, weeks, or even months for an appointment with an overworked physician. However, the hospital and its associated clinics are usually even more likely to create feelings of alienation. The patient is usually admitted to the new and strange hospital environment when illness has already rendered him relatively helpless and attacked his self-concept. In this setting, the patient feels normless, which means he has no set of standards to which to relate his behavior. Many of his usual standards of personal conduct —including bodily modesty, personal self-care, pursuit of useful activities, and self-direction in his personal affairs—no longer apply. He realizes this but has difficulty responding as he is now expected to. He is not permitted to help himself, but how much help is he permitted to ask of hospital personnel? Are there still rules of modesty he is expected to obey? If so, which and how? He is expected to report his symptoms, but how freely may he do so without being accused of complaining? He is cut off from those to whom he usually expresses his fear and despair but how freely may he speak about these to hospital personnel? These and many other questions perplex and stress the patient as he attempts to meet the expectations of hospital personnel in his new role of hospital patient.

Powerlessness is another aspect of alienation commonly engendered by the hospital setting. He has little or no control over what happens to him. Every detail of his life is regulated by doctor's orders or hospital regulations. He is admitted and discharged at the will of the authorities and must conform to hospital regulations and arrangements about meals, medications, diet, and visitors.

A sense of meaninglessness often numbs hospital patients. The reasons for the regulations and procedures in a bureaucratically organized hospital, and much of his medical treatment as well, may remain obscure to the patient. He is incapable of engaging in many of the activities and social relationships which lent meaning to his life or is prevented from doing so by the restrictions imposed by the hospital. Alone in a sterile atmosphere isolated from friends and family, subjected to strange and often painful procedures, life itself may become meaningless to the patient.

Self-estrangement is also sometimes part of the hospital experience. A sense of unreality may pervade the self when one is deprived of one's own clothing and other possessions and of the support of customary relationships. Hospital personnel do not treat an individual as he is accustomed to being treated, and in the role of patient, he is not in a position to exhibit many of the personal qualities and capacities which ordinarily elicit responses that support his sense of self.

The interviewer in the hospital situation has his own set of problems. The private physician making hospital rounds usually feels less at home than in his own office. Given the changing roles of physicians in hospitals he may be engaged in role conflicts with the hospital administration or the burgeoning staff of new health personnel. He must adjust his practice to the hospital's bureaucratic procedures, and his practice is more open to the scrutiny of his colleagues than it is when he is in his office. The staff physician, the nurses, and other personnel may feel more comfortable in the hospital, but they also have many problems which make effective interviewing difficult. Hospitals are usually understaffed which means that health professionals are tightly scheduled and overworked. Large teaching hospitals are likely to foster segmented care and divided professional responsibility through their highly specialized services making it difficult for any single professional to have the rapport with a patient that develops with successive interviews.

The immediate situation provided in a hospital is likely to be unfavorable for an effective interview. The patient is more frequently than not in a ward or shared room, and hospital personnel or visitors may interrupt the interview. The patient is usually in bed while the interviewer is clothed and mobile. In this situation, some interviewers stand at the foot of the bed, some at the side of the bed, and some sit on or near the bed while talking to the patient. In each case, the effect on the interview varies. The physical distance from the patient has an effect on the emotional distance; they vary directly with each other. The standing physician speaking with a patient who is lying down creates a status difference that reduces communication. The physician who is sitting and close enough to touch the patient will be helping to create an atmosphere that is supportive and that encourages communication.

Each health care delivery system defines the task of the health professional with respect to the patient's care somewhat differently. This definition affects the information to be obtained in the interview and the quality of the relationship formed with the patient. In general, the larger and more complex the health care system and the more specialized the services provided by the individual health worker, the more difficult it is to provide continuity and coordination of health services and the more alienative is the process of health care. The scope of the interview will ordinarily be defined by the nature of the service to be performed. The laboratory technician about to draw blood will probably conduct a brief interview obtaining information immediately relevant to the procedure, putting the patient at ease, and, if required, relieving his anxiety about the procedure. The more comprehensive the professional's responsibility for the patient, the more comprehensive the interview required. Health care systems in which the patient is seen many times by different individuals in circumscribed interviews contribute to feelings of alienation.

REFERENCES

1. Goffman, E., *Strategic Interaction*. Philadelphia: University of Pennsylvania Press, 1969.
2. Parsons, T., *The Social System*. New York: The Free Press, 1951.
3. Clark, M., *Health in the Mexican-American Culture*. Los Angeles and Berkeley: University of California Press, 1970.
4. Greenwood, E., "Attributes of a Profession," *Social Work*, 2:45-55, 1957.
5. Gross, E., *Work and Society*. New York: Crowell, 1958, pp. 77-82.
6. Goode, W. J., "Encroachment, Charlatanism, and the Emerging Professions: Psychology, Sociology, and Medicine," *American Sociological Review*, 25:903, 1960.
7. Hall, R. H., *Occupations and the Social Structure*. Englewood Cliffs, N.J.: Prentice-Hall, 1969.
8. Freidson, E., *Profession of Medicine*. New York: Dodd, Mead, 1970.

9. Freidson, E., Ibid.
10. Coleman, J. S., E. Katz, and H. Menzel, *Medical Innovation, A Diffusion Study*. Indianapolis: Bobbs-Merrill, 1966.
11. Coleman, J. S., E. Katz, and H. Menzel, Ibid., p. 71.
12. King, S. H., Ibid.
13. Schulman, S., "Basic Functional Roles in Nursing: Mother Surrogate and Healer," in E. G. Jaco (ed.), *Patients, Physicians and Illness*. Glencoe, Ill.: The Free Press, 1958, pp. 528-537.
14. King, S. H., Ibid.
15. Fink, A. E., C. W. Anderson, and M. B. Conover, *The Field of Social Work*. New York: Holt, Rinehart and Winston. 5th Ed., 1968, p. 275.
16. Fink, A. E., et al., Ibid. p. 276.
17. Fink, et al., Ibid. pp. 283-284.
18. Hall, R. H., Ibid.
19. Simmons, O., "Implications of Social Class for Public Health," in E. G. Jaco (ed.), *Patients, Physicians and Illness*. Glencoe, Ill.: The Free Press, 1958, pp. 107-112.
20. Paul, B. D., *Health, Culture and Community*. New York: Russell Sage, 1955.
21. Seeman, M., and J. W. Evans, "Alienation and Learning in a Hospital Setting," *American Sociological Review*, 27:772-782, 1962.

11

MEDICAL QUESTIONNAIRES AND AUTOMATED DATA GATHERING

1 INTRODUCTION

This book has emphasized the personal role of the health care professional as an observer, particularly as he interacts with the patient during an interview. Although the physician's interviewing is an essential medical skill, it should be recognized that useful medical data can be collected in other ways. These auxiliary data gathering techniques do not substitute for the important clinical care process by which a doctor-patient relationship is formed, a unique feature of the personal interview. Nevertheless, they may provide important data for a variety of purposes. They may supplement the personal interview or serve in situations where a therapeutic relationship is not required. We will examine in this chapter some of these ancillary modes of data gathering and their uses. Finally, we will consider some of the uses of rapid automatic data processing methods in use at present and of promise in the future.

Use of Trained Interviewers

Certain kinds of medically useful information are commonly collected by non-physician health workers and by clerical persons in many health care settings. A logical outgrowth of this practice has been the training in some medical centers of non-physician interviewers who obtain a basic description of the patient's illness. The information is used to refer the patient properly within a clinic, for example, or to provide starting information for the physician who will care for that patient. With the current emphasis on development of paramedical personnel to extend the health care system of the United States, we believe this practice will become widespread. Non-physician interviewers can be trained to gather information in much the same fashion as the physician should be trained. Their interpretation of what the patient says, however, must be limited. The data should be recorded in as close to their original form as possible.

2 QUESTIONNAIRES

Non-physician interviewers have been trained to administer a predetermined program of questions designed to elicit specific information in addition to that which the patient has volunteered. These question programs can be quite detailed and time-consuming, with branched subsets of questions to be administered if the patient responds positively to a general question. A great deal of information may be gathered, but the affective context of the patient's response to questions is commonly lost to those who review this information. If the physician and interviewer have a well-defined relationship and effective communication, more non-verbal information can be salvaged. Programs of questions should be carefully chosen if they are used, and each item periodically examined for its productivity.[1] Too often, more or less traditional questions are asked without evaluation of their usefulness.

Use of Ancillary Data Gathering Methods

Ancillary data gathering methods may be characterized as interactive and non-interactive. An interactive method implies the presence and participation of a human observer who is capable of directing the data gathering process to a limited degree and observing the patient's non-verbal affective responses as he deals with the various topics. In this respect, interactive data gathering by a third person follows the general model of the interview. It differs, of course, in that it imposes a rather rigidly organized structure on the data-gathering process.

Non-interactive methods discard the observational kinds of data in favor of greater economy of time. Structured data-gathering methods may be designed to supplement information about the patient's primary problems obtained by an interview, as in the case of a psychological test. Or, they may complement the basic information by filling in more general background information unrelated, or only indirectly related, to the patient's immediate problems. An example of the latter would be the use of a questionnaire to obtain information about the patient's past medical history and what is usually called the "review of systems."

Computer administered questionnaires with highly branched programs of questions are sometimes spoken of as interactive, since the machine responds in programed fashion to the patient's responses to the question. This is not interaction in the human sense, of course, which involves the emotional and intellectual response of one person to another.

Use of Questionnaires

Self-administered questionnaires are most common and have the advantage of allowing the patient to proceed at his own pace. But they do have disadvantages. If at all complex, they require high levels of linguistic skill and attention from the patient. This may be difficult or impossible for certain patients, particularly those who are quite ill or psychologically disturbed. If the questionnaire involves branching, that is, administration of a subset of questions when a given response is positive, the patient may have difficulty following the directions. The questionnaire itself may be bulky and formidable in appearance, leading the patient to "give up." Nevertheless, for certain purposes, such as screening health examinations for apparently well patients, self-administered questionnaires of careful design may be useful.

Questionnaires may be designed with yes-no and multiple-choice items so as to elicit a restricted range of responses. Such questionnaires are usually employed as screening devices where the object is to select out persons who have an increased probability of having a specific disorder. A high number of false positives can be expected in using such an instrument. These people must be further categorized by more detailed study. Ideally, screening questionnaires should have a low rate of false negatives, that is, they should rarely fail to identify the individual who has the condition being sought.

If more definitive and more general data about an individual patient are to be acquired by questionnaire, a broader range of responses must be obtained. This may be done by requiring the patient to fill in a blank space in his own words in response to the question. While useful to a physician who reads and interprets the questionnaire, such responses are not yet amenable to automated data processing. Branching questionnaires, with subsets of questions arranged in a hierarchial fashion, provide a second approach to the problem of obtaining more definitive data from an individual patient. Here larger numbers of logically related questions may be asked with a restricted number of responses permitted for each question. The nature of the response at each point determines the next question to be posed.

Administration of Questionnaires by Computer

Questionnaires with high levels of branching become very large, complex, and difficult to follow when presented on paper. Computers can be programed to administer such questionnaires and to record and process the patient's responses.[2, 3, 4, 5, 6] The problems of computer administration of questionnaires largely relate to the input devices that must be used by the patient to enter his responses into the machine. Typewriters and other keyboard devices are difficult to use without experience. Cathode ray tube displays with a limited number of buttons to press or touch points seem to be the most useful technology developed to date. Again, the care with which the questions are designed and assessed will determine the value of the results of computer-based questionnaires. The computer provides only a technology of administration and will not turn a fundamentally poor set of questions into a useful data gathering device.

Computers can collate, relate and print out the patient's responses to a questionnaire. The printout can be devised in a way that provides a narrative which reads much like the historical part of a medical record. Computers can also keep cumulative records of large numbers of patient responses for research purposes, or for future reevaluation. Permanent records can also be stored in these machines.

Standardized Tests

Many highly developed and standardized psychological tests, such as the Minnesota Multiphasic Personality Inventory,[7] are in the form of questionnaires. In clinical medicine such tests will produce specific information about a limited aspect of the patient's current status. They should be viewed as ancillary diagnostic tools to be used in much the same way as laboratory, radiological, and clinical physiological studies are used in elucidating and evaluating a patient's problems. They should be employed after a general clinical study of the patient has suggested a specific structured test will be useful in clarifying the nature of a problem that has been identified.

Some Problems of Questionnaires

The most general problem with questionnaires is their inflexibility. Development of more sophisticated computer-based methods, possibly with some element of human interaction, may reduce this problem markedly. We have already mentioned the limitations imposed by illiteracy and limited linguistic ability of the patient, and by serious acute or psychiatric illness. Non-interactive questionnaires are usually unsuccessful with patients of low intelligence.

Patients must also be well motivated to provide useful data. Some patients may reject questionnaires as evidence of a lack of interest in them or they may feel that such an approach is clearly irrelevant to their problems. The American public is rapidly approaching utter boredom, intolerance, and unresponsiveness to questionnaires in general. If a specific questionnaire gains widespread acceptance, the patient may be confronted with it several times as he receives medical care in different places. He becomes worried about the consistency of his responses and the interpretations that may be made of discrepancies. This may inhibit his responsiveness to all data-gathering efforts.

Finally, we should recognize that bias can be introduced into the data obtained from a patient by questionnaire methods in the same ways that it can be introduced by personal interviews. These biases can be of content, based upon the nature of the questions asked, and of sequence, based upon the order of the questions. Indeed, it seems probable that a highly skilled interviewer would be less likely to introduce biases than most questionnaires would be. If a patient is to be both interviewed and given a questionnaire, it seems reasonable to carry out the procedures in this order. Unfortunately, the order is usually reversed in practice, since the aim of most data gathering methods not based upon interviewing is to save physician time by "predigesting" a certain base of information for him.

3 USES OF COMPUTERS

Computer Based Processing of Medical Information

Much has been written in the last decade about the uses of computers to support the practice of medicine and facilitate the distribution of medical care. Two aspects of this technology deserve brief mention here, because they relate to the general problems of data gathering, record keeping, and medical problem solving. These are computerized data retrieval and computer-assisted medical diagnosis. For those interested in a detailed discussion of the medical uses of computers, the books by Ledley and by Jacquez should be consulted.[6, 7]

Computerized Data Retrieval

Many kinds of medical records are already being handled effectively by computer techniques in a variety of institutional settings. These records commonly include basic identification information, fiscal and administrative data, laboratory records, orders for drugs and other services, and in some cases the output of patient monitoring devices. Properly organized, a computer can serve to gather, record, store, and deliver most kinds of information in a variety of output formats at the places where the data will be used. At a more powerful level of organization, a machine can serve as the fundamental element of a health information system; this implies programed data collection, delivery of segments of data to the appropriate places, and carrying out automatically the appropriate related transactions. Systems in which computers handle all the information of a hospital or of even larger area-wide health care organizations have been designed and are under evaluation. It seems probable that the physician of the future and his institutions will have substantial support from computer-based information systems.

Computer Assisted Medical Diagnosis

The advent of computers with their power and speed in solving numerical and logical problems very early led to investigation of their usefulness in assisting or simulating the diagnostic problem-solving process of the physician.[10] Although the practical results of these efforts have been of limited value thus far, this work has served to focus attention on the important question of how physicians arrive at diagnoses. It is surprising how little is known of the high level mental processes involved in this activity. Important knowledge is now appearing which may help to design better ways to learn these skills.

Useful computer programs have been developed to solve limited, highly describable diagnostic problems which deal with discrete, quantitative data, for example, the interpretation of electrocardiograms or the evaluation of the output of cardiovascular physiological monitors.[11] These programs will reproduce the results of the equivalent human mental process even though they may not simulate that process. It is probable that a number of useful programs of this type will soon be available. Physicians must learn to use these aids in the same way other diagnostic assistance is employed. The results must be evaluated in light of the patient's full clinical picture.

More general computer programs for medical diagnosis have been attempted with less success. These have been of two main types. In the first, the computer serves mainly to remind the physician of essentially all the diagnostic possibilities compatible with a given set of available data. A second, more ambitious approach attempts to resolve a base of requisite data into the diagnosis or diagnoses of highest probability. Refinements of this approach may also indicate relative statistical probabilities and courses of action which will distinguish between the several possibilities. Neither approach is yet entirely workable in the setting of medical practice. The first may have more immediate prospects of utility, since physicians commonly miss diagnoses because they fail to think of a rare possibility. Some aspects of the second approach may also be available soon to aid the physician who does not know how to proceed in separating alternative possible diagnoses by critical tests. When all of the necessary data are available to make a diagnosis, the diagnosis itself is frequently apparent.

Some Problems in the Medical Uses of Computers

Computers deal best with information in easily accessible numerical form. Data in verbal form are storable in computers but as yet are difficult to analyze and manipulate when compared to numerical data. The accessibility of the primary data to the computer is commonly poor, resulting in slow inputs, a condition referred to as "input bound." By contrast, the capability of machines to compute, sort, transfer and transform data is commonly many orders of magnitude faster and more efficient than the processes by which the machine first captures the information. Biomedical computing would be greatly facilitated by faster, more efficient data input techniques.

Certain kinds of information which may be apparent to an interviewer and of great diagnostic value are difficult or impossible to capture in a form usable in computers. These are the data obtained from one's human interaction with the patient, empathic reactions, evaluations of gestures, facial expressions, and other observations of affect. A spontaneous clutching gesture made to the precordium when the patient is talking about chest pain reveals much to the trained physician observer who is familiar with angina pectoris. As yet, such information is impossible to encode for computer recording and processing purposes without the use of a human observer.

It is obvious that even an efficient and powerful computer-based information gathering and processing system still will not substitute for the physician's relationship with the patient through which he should exert profound therapeutic effects. Therefore, the physician must spend at least a minimum amount of time talking with the patient about his illness and its problems, during which he is also gathering data. Although computers may assist the physician and save some time for him, they cannot be substituted for him unless the practice of medicine is to change radically in the future.

The Future

Enthusiasts have predicted functions for computers in medicine which border on science fiction. It does not seem unreasonable to look forward to the day when there will be some interactive mode of patient, physician, and computer data gathering with retrieval, distribution, and processing of the data for problem-solving purposes as a functional part of a technologically advanced health care system. A little further imagination brings us to computers capable of learning from their own experience as well as accepting instructions from an external programer. Image-processing techniques may capture data in pictorial or graphic form and provide automated interpretations of these data. Indeed, it is not too difficult to foresee the day when substantial numbers of physicians will also be trained as systems scientists; they will then have to learn the skill of "interviewing" in the arcane languages of complex machine systems which work for them.

4 FURTHER DEVELOPMENT OF THE PROBLEM-ORIENTED MEDICAL RECORD

In Chapter 5 we referred to several variations of the problem-oriented medical record introduced by Weed. The example provided in that chapter is a blend of the classical clinical record and the full application of Weed's approach. Such compromises have been adapted in a number of medical centers in an effort to present both "the problems" and "the whole picture" of the patient in written records, while still adhering to the basic techniques of the P.O.R.

If medical records are to be under truly powerful control of computers, the data entered into the system must first be identified by designating the problems to which they are pertinent. At present computers are unable to carry out this basic data sorting, but the methods of context analysis may permit machines to sort raw data some day. If all the relevant data are assigned to an identified problem from the time the record is first created, a computer will be able to retrieve specifically all the data about that problem regardless of when it was obtained. Alternatively, it can retrieve and reassemble a cross-sectional view of all the patient's problems at any point in time or over a defined time span. Obviously, other options for data retrieval, reassembly, and delivery exist once the data are under this basic control. These comments relate to systems in which the information is stored in electromagnetic form within the computer itself, or when they are stored in an optical system, such as microfiche, with the retrieval of the cards carried out by a computer controlled opticomechanical system.

As an example of a completely developed problem-oriented record which might be appropriate for a computer-based data control system, we again present the medical record of Chapter 5. We emphasize that the P.O.R. in this format is also entirely compatible with a "paper based" record-keeping system; as we see it, this format is required for maximal utility of automated medical data handling systems, whether for retrieval or for analytical purposes.

Records in the fully problem-oriented format still present a number of problems not yet resolved by widely accepted conventions. The record presented here varies in certain ways from the conventions recommended by Weed. What to do with data which are not assignable to a current problem, such as certain social data, normal physical findings, color of eyes or hair, is one problem. These data must be recorded since they may be very pertinent to some new problem that may develop in the future when it is important to know that certain findings have changed. We have chosen to record most of these data under an "Unassigned Data Base" and in the patient profile. Note that certain data are recorded both here and under a titled problem. Other data might have been recorded in several places also, if they are pertinent to more than one problem and also part of that general picture of the person provided by the patient profile.

Also note that the master problem list is different in this example. The record of what the patient is told by the physician is not included under the initial problem formulations but could well have been added. Finally, the progress notes are not repeated since they would be the same as those given in the P.O.R. of Chapter 5.

MICHIGAN STATE UNIVERSITY HEALTH CENTER
East Lansing, Michigan 48823

CLINICAL RECORD

Date & Time | Patient Name: Miss Mary Blank | Unit Record No. 16711

MASTER PROBLEM LIST

Date & Time	Problem Number		Outcome
1/10/72	1	Uterine Bleeding	
1/10/72	2	Weight Loss	Retitled 1/11/72
1/10/72	3	Arthritis	
1/10/72	4	Depression	
1/10/72	5	Anemia	
1/11/72	2	Diabetes Mellitus	Formerly titled "weight loss"
1/11/72	4	Adjustment reaction of adult life (grief reaction)	Formerly titled "depression"

Prepared by: ______________________ Staff title/Student status ______________________

MICHIGAN STATE UNIVERSITY HEALTH CENTER
East Lansing, Michigan 48823
CLINICAL RECORD

Date & Time — Patient Name: Miss Mary Blank — Unit Record No. 16711

INITIAL EVALUATION

1/10/72 9:00 a.m.

This patient is a 42 year old single white woman, a law office secretary, who was brought to the hospital by a friend who called for her this morning to take her to work and found her still in bed. The patient has no voluntary complaints, but on questioning first states that "my menstrual periods are too heavy," and also indicates that she is weak and losing weight. She is reserved, quiet, and seems sad.

PROBLEM #1 Vaginal bleeding. Historical: This woman noticed increasingly heavy menstrual flow about 8 months ago. Periods have lasted 7 to 9 days during which she daily soaked through several standard pads. The periods were normally timed, without discomfort or other notable symptoms.

Three months ago, a normally timed period started and lasted 12 days. She passed clots on the second, third and fourth days which she spent in bed. Since this period, she has had intermittent vaginal bleeding, every 3 to 5 days, varying in amount from slight spotting to enough to require 2 to 3 pads daily, lasting a day or two at a time. She thinks she has had one normally timed period, starting about December 5, 1971. This was also heavy and prolonged. She did not seek medical care because she felt this problem was due to "change of life." She has had no pregnancies.

Two days ago, in the late afternoon, she began to feel much worse with the onset of nausea, anorexia, and greatly increased weakness. She has been somewhat somnolent since.

Findings: No generalized hemorrhagic manifestations of skin or mucous membranes.

Abdomen: There is a slight mid-abdominal distension and tympany. No organs or masses are palpable. There is distinct tenderness and some guarding on deep suprapubic palpation.

Pelvic Examination: The external genitalia are normal. The introitus is virginal, and speculum and manual examination were unsatisfactory. The vaginal mucosa appears normal, as does the cervix. There was no bleeding. There was tenderness anteriorly on palpation. The uterus was thought to be 3 to 4 times normal size and somewhat irregular in contour.

Rectal Examination: Confirms findings of pelvic exam. There are no rectal abnormalities.

Prepared by: ____________________ Staff title/Student status ____________________

MICHIGAN STATE UNIVERSITY HEALTH CENTER
East Lansing, Michigan 48823
CLINICAL RECORD

Date & Time

Patient Name: Miss Mary Blank Unit Record No. 16711

Formulation: The source of the vaginal bleeding appears to be the uterus. The uterine enlargement suggests the presence of a tumor. Distinction between a benign tumor, and an endometrial cancer cannot be made on the basis of available data. It is possible, but unlikely, that she has a bleeding diathesis on the basis of the aspirin she has taken. There is no evidence of a generalized hemorrhagic disorder.

Plan: Diagnostic - Gyn consultation for exam under anesthesia; pap smear and possibly biopsy of D & C.
Therapeutic - none needed at present.

PROBLEM #2 Weight loss. Historical: She felt quite well until about 4 months ago, when she began to experience increasing fatigue, decreased exercise tolerance, and weight loss of about 14 pounds. She feels her appetite has increased if anything and she has eaten regularly. She has not felt tremulous or noted heat intolerance. Nor has she noted excessive thirst or increased urine volume, although she habitually urinates frequently. A paternal aunt, age 50, has diabetes. She thinks her paternal grandmother also had diabetes.

She describes her diet as well balanced with meals precisely timed. Weight has averaged 124 lbs. over past 10 years varying only a few pounds. Highest weight, 130 in 1952.

She has not noted vision changes. She has never had a goiter or any evidence of thyroid disease; her voice is unchanged.

Findings: Present weight 110 lbs., ht. 66". The skin is normal except for some loss of turgor suggesting dehydration. Eyes are normal except for a moderate narrowing of the arteries and some increased tortuosity. Vessels - brachial arteries feel normal. All pulses are normally palpable. Neck - the thyroid gland is palpable, smooth, and normal in size. There is no tremor. The urine shows 2+ glucose and 2+ acetone.

Formulation: The weight loss could be compatible with a malignant uterine tumor, although there is no evidence of metastasis or extension. The glycosuria raises the possibility of diabetes, although she is not in apparent acidosis. Hyperthyroidism or other metabolic or gastrointestinal causes of weight loss seem unlikely.

Plan: Diagnostic - Blood sugar, BUN, and electrolyte determinations stat.
Therapeutic - Start IV fluids and await results above.

Prepared by: Staff title/Student status

MICHIGAN STATE UNIVERSITY HEALTH CENTER
East Lansing, Michigan 48823
CLINICAL RECORD

Date & Time — Patient Name: Miss Mary Blank — Unit Record No. 16711

PROBLEM #3 Arthritis. Historical: She has had intermittent joint swelling, pain and stiffness in the hands, wrists, and shoulders, as well as occasionally in other joints for the past six years. She has had little joint deformity, but intermittently takes as many as 12 aspirin tablets a day for pain. This was diagnosed as rheumatoid arthritis at the University of Michigan Clinics in 1968. She has been taking aspirin in doses of 6 to 12 tablets a day for the last 2 months. Occasionally, she takes a proprietary "extra strength" product, the name of which she cannot recall now.

Findings: The proximal interphalangeal joints of both hands show thickening, slight limitation of motion on flexion with tapering of the fingers. The skin of the fingers is smooth, but thin and supple. The right wrist is also affected. The remaining joints appear normal and exhibit normal mobility.

Formulation: Probably rheumatoid disease, with little evidence of activity at the present.

Plans: Diagnostic - Request information from University of Michigan Arthritis Clinic.
Therapeutic - No medication for present.

PROBLEM #4 Depression. Historical: This woman lived with her mother who died of metastatic carcinoma of the colon in November of 1969 at age 61. She feels a mixture of sadness, relief, and guilt over her sense of relief following her mother's death. She has had recurrent insomnia and feelings of sadness and hopelessness, and she cried daily for a month after her mother died.

She has felt somewhat better from this point of view in the last few months. She still has occasional periods of sadness and crying. She has been able to keep up with her demanding position as office manager in the legal office where she has worked for over 20 years.

During the last 5 years, she has had headaches 1 to 3 times weekly characterized by a feeling of tightness in the back of her head and neck and head pain which radiates forward bilaterally from this region. She has no visual or other aura or related phenomena. The headaches are precipitated by fatigue, excessive work stress and frustration. They are promptly relieved by rest and aspirin.

Prepared by: ____________ Staff title/Student status ____________

MICHIGAN STATE UNIVERSITY HEALTH CENTER
East Lansing, Michigan 48823
CLINICAL RECORD

Date & Time | Patient Name: Miss Mary Blank | Unit Record No. 16711

Observation: Her mental status evaluation revealed the following: Appearance and behavior - quiet, reserved, pale, colorless, responds slowly, looks sad, never smiles. Speech - soft voice; clear but brief answers; never elaborates unless encouraged. Mood - looks depressed. Admits to feeling "blue." States this has improved recently. Thought content - still grieving for her mother. No suicidal ideas. No evidence of psychotic thought disorder. Orientation - clear.

Formulation: This woman probably has a reactive or situational depression following the death of her mother. She has historical evidence of tension headaches. Her social background suggests a high level of isolation, but she has functioned well in her job, without decompensation.

Plan: Diagnostic - Patient will be evaluated on medical psychiatric rounds tomorrow.
Therapeutic - Dependent upon consultant's recommendation. We will not give her any anti-depressant drugs at present.

PROBLEM #5 Anemia. Historical: She has had excessive blood loss as noted in problem #1. She feels she has become increasingly pale, and she has taken a proprietary iron tablet twice daily for several months. She has not been known to be anemic in the past and there is no familial history of anemia.

Observations: Pallor of skin and mucosae. No significant lymphodenopathy. Spleen is not palpable.

Hematology Laboratory Findings: Hematocrit 30%, Hgb. 8.8 gm.%, WBC 11,000/cu.mm. Differential count: Polys. 60%, Band forms 4%, Eosinophils 1%, Basophils 0%, Monocytes 7%, Lymphocytes 28%. The red cells show hypochromia, anisocytosis, microcytosis, and polychromasia. The leukocytes are normal in appearance. Platelets are present in normal numbers and appear normal.

Formulation: The blood picture appears to be that of iron deficiency anemia, probably due to uterine blood loss. There is no evidence of a primary blood dyscrasia, nor of metastatic tumor in bone marrow.

Plan: Diagnostic - Reticulocyte count, red cell indices. Bone marrow examination for iron stores. Stools for blood.
Therapeutic - If low iron stores, administer ferrous sulphate in increasing doses, starting with 0.2 gm. p.o. with largest meal.

Prepared by: ______________________ Staff title/Student status ______________________

MICHIGAN STATE UNIVERSITY HEALTH CENTER
East Lansing, Michigan 48823

CLINICAL RECORD

Date & Time

Patient Name: Miss Mary Blank Unit Record No. 16711

PATIENT PROFILE: The patient is a rather tall, thin, pale woman who looks somewhat older than her stated age. She looks both chronically and acutely ill. She responds precisely to all questions, but somewhat slowly, without apparent emotion. She interacts minimally on interview and examination.

Miss Blank was born on January 5, 1930, on a farm south of Lansing, Michigan, and grew up there. After high school, she studied fine arts at Michigan State University for two years. She commuted from home and earned most of her expenses as a stenographer. After her father's death, she stopped attending college, moved to Lansing with her mother and began to work as a secretary in a legal office. She describes her mother as a dependent, inadequate person who was recurrently depressed after her father's death. She speaks without overt resentment of "having devoted my entire life to mother." She describes herself as a lonely, isolated person with few friends and little social life; she is absorbed by her job. The patient has never married. She was the only child of parents both now deceased. Her mother died in November 1969 of metastatic carcinoma of the colon at age 61, as noted in problem #4.

UNASSIGNED DATA BASE: Her parents were both of English origin. There is no history of familial diseases, including hemorrhagic disorders or anemia.

She has enjoyed good health in general. She had measles, mumps, chicken pox, and acute tonsillitis as a child. Her only surgical operation was a tonsillectomy at age 9 which was uneventful. She has not had other hemorrhagic manifestations in the past or with the present illness.

Does not drink or smoke and has not in the past. Takes no drugs regularly except aspirin and related products.

Allergies: None known.

Eyes: She wears glasses.

Mouth: She has lost both lower right molar teeth and they are unreplaced.

Skin: She has had no evidence of excessive bruising or petechial hemorrhages. She has had no pigmentary changes, or changes in hair distribution or characteristics.

PHYSICAL EXAMINATION: Pulse 95 BPM; Temp. 38°C p.o.; Resp. 19/min.; BP 108/70 Right arm reclining; Ht. 66", Wt. 110 lbs.

Prepared by: Staff title/Student status

MICHIGAN STATE UNIVERSITY HEALTH CENTER
East Lansing, Michigan 48823
CLINICAL RECORD

Date & Time | Patient Name: Miss Mary Blank | Unit Record No. 16711

Ears, Nose, Throat: Normal. Mouth: The tongue is heavily coated. The mucosae appear moderately dehydrated and pale. Lower right molar teeth missing. The remaining teeth are in good repair, but the gingivae appear red, slightly swollen, and retracted around the canine and lateral incisors in the lower jaw.

Neck: Normal.

Lymphatic System: A soft 1/2 cm. node is palpable high in the left axilla. No other notable glands.

Chest: Normal configuration. Respiration is somewhat deeper than normal and slightly accelerated.

Lungs: Clear in all areas.

Heart: Normal rhythm. Tachycardia is persistent. Heart size, shape, and sounds are normal.

Peripheral Vessels: Veins and venous pressure appear to be normal. No edema.

Breasts: Small, showing signs of recent weight loss. No abnormalities.

Neurological: Within normal limits.

Urinalysis: pH 5.0, specific gravity 1.035, cloudy, dark amber. Glucose 2+, Acetone 2+, protein Tr, Micro: Rare WBC. Gram stain - few gram neg. rods.

Prepared by: ______________________ Staff title/Student status

REFERENCES

1. Brodman, K., A. J. Edmann, Jr., I. Lorge, and H. G. Wolff, "The Cornell Medical Index," *JAMA*, 140:530, 1949.
2. Slack, W. V., and L. J. Van Cura, "Computer-based Patient Interviewing," Part I. *Postgraduate Medicine*, 43:68-74, 1968; Part II, ibid., 43:115-120, 1968.
3. Slack, W. V., G. P. Hicks, C. E. Reed, and L. J. Van Cura, "A Computer-based Medical History System," *New England Journal of Medicine*, 247:194-198, 1966.
4. Slack, W. V., and L. J. Van Cura, "Patient Reaction to Computer-based Medical Interviewing, *Comput. Biomed. Res.*, 1:527-531, 1968.
5. Mayne, J. G., M. J. Martin, G. W. Morrow, Jr., R. M. Turner, and B. L. Hisey, "A Health Questionnaire Based on Paper-and-Pencil Medium Individualized and Produced by Computer, I. Technique," *JAMA*, 208:2060-2063, 1969.
6. Martin, M. J., J. G. Mayne, W. F. Taylor, and M. N. Swenson, "A Health Questionnaire Based on Paper-and-Pencil Medium Individualized and Produced by Computer, II. Testing and Evaluation," *JAMA*, 208:2064-2068, 1969.
7. Rowe, H. P., W. M. Swenson, P. Mataya, C. E. McCarthy, J. S. Pearson, F. R. Keating, and S. R. Hathaway, "Symposium on Automation Technics in Personality Assessment," *Proc. Staff. Mtg. Mayo Clinic*, 37:61-82, 1962.
8. Taylor, T. R., "*The Principles of Medical Computing*" Oxford: Blackwell Scientific Publications, Ltd., 1967.
9. Jacquez, John A., "Algorithmic Diagnosis: A Review with Emphasis on Bayesian Methods," in J. A. Jacquez (Ed.), *Computer Diagnosis and Diagnostic Methods*. Springfield, Ill.: Charles C Thomas, 1972.
10. Gorry, G. A., "Prospects for Computer-aided Diagnosis," *New England Journal of Medicine*, 281:101-102, 1969.
11. Caceres, C. A., and L. S. Dreifus (Eds.), *Clinical Electrocardiography and Computers*. New York, Academic Press, 1970.

INDEX